Radiographic Interpretation for the Dental Hygienist

Joen Iannucci Haring, DDS, MS

Assistant Professor
Section of Diagnostic Services
The Ohio State University
College of Dentistry
Columbus, Ohio

Laura Jansen, RDH, MS

Clinical Associate Professor
Department of Dental Ecology
School of Dentistry
The University of North Carolina at Chapel Hill
Chapel Hill, North Carolina

SAUNDERS

An Imprint of Elsevier

SAUNDERS
An Imprint of Elsevier
The Curtis Center
Independence Square West
Philadelphia, PA 19106

Library of Congress Cataloging-in-Publication Data

Haring, Joen Iannucci.
    Radiographic interpretation for the dental hygienist/Joen
Iannucci Haring, Laura Jansen Lind.
        p.   cm.
    Includes index.
    ISBN-13: 978-0-7216-3704-4   ISBN-10: 0-7216-3704-3
    1. Teeth—Radiography.   2. Teeth—Diseases—Diagnosis.   I. Lind,
Laura Jansen.   II. Title.
    [DNLM: 1. Radiography, Dental.   WN 230 H281r]
RK309.437   1993
617.6'07572—dc20
DNLM/DLC   92-49496

ISBN-13: 978-0-7216-3704-4
ISBN-10: 0-7216-3704-3

Radiographic Interpretation for the Dental Hygienist

Printed in the United States of America.

Last digit is the print number: 13   12

To my family and friends
who have encouraged me
throughout my career, and,

To my steadfast supporters:
my husband—Robert S. Haring,
my father—Angelo J. Iannucci, and
my grandfather—Angelo M. Iannucci.

—JIH

To the educators who have influenced me:

my parents—Margaret E. and Leonard C. Jansen
my mentors—Margot L. VanDis and Richard C. O'Brien

To my family and friends, who are the best part of my life.

—LJ

PREFACE

Dental radiographs are a necessary component of comprehensive patient care and enable the practitioner to identify many conditions that may otherwise go undetected. Interpretation, or the ability to read what is revealed by a radiograph, is an essential part of the diagnostic process. The dental hygienist can play a vital role in the interpretation of dental radiographs. The purpose of *Radiographic Interpretation for the Dental Hygienist* is to provide the reader with a comprehensive and well-organized overview of radiographic interpretation.

Radiographic Interpretation for the Dental Hygienist provides the reader with a logical, step-by-step approach to the interpretation of dental radiographs. Topics include the importance of dental radiographs, film mounting and viewing; descriptive terminology; normal anatomic structures seen on periapical and panoramic films; identification of restorations, dental materials and foreign objects; dental caries; periodontal disease; trauma, pulpal and periapical lesions; and film exposure, processing and technique errors.

What makes *Radiographic Interpretation for the Dental Hygienist* unique? The material presented in this book is *not* typically found in one textbook; instead, it is usually found in bits and pieces in textbooks on oral radiology, oral pathology, human anatomy, dental anatomy, periodontology and restorative dentistry. In this text, information found in a variety of books has been combined and organized into one easy-to-use reference source.

Each chapter in *Radiographic Interpretation for the Dental Hygienist* includes a list of objectives to help the reader focus on important aspects of the material presented. At the beginning of each chapter, key words are listed; each key word is highlighted in boldface as it is introduced in the text. Quiz questions are included at the end of each chapter. Numerous line drawings, photographs and radiographs are used throughout the text to illustrate examples of each topic discussed. Simple and straightforward explanations and examples are used to foster comprehension and retention of concepts presented. A glossary of over 200 terms is included at the end of the text.

We wish to express our gratitude to William L. Lind, DDS, for his editorial assistance in preparation of this manuscript. We wish to acknowledge Carl M. Allen, DDS, MSD, and Robert M. Jaynes, DDS, MS, for their contribution of radiographs, John G. Snyder and John W. Snyder for their photographic expertise, Susan M. Bauchmoyer, RDH, BS, for her contributions and support and Anna Layton and Gail Snewin for their technical assistance. Most importantly, we wish to thank our husbands, Robert S. Haring, DDS, MS, and William L. Lind, DDS, for their encouragement, patience and continuous support.

—Joen Iannucci Haring, DDS, MS
—Laura Jansen Lind, RDH, MS

TABLE OF CONTENTS

CHAPTER ONE

The Importance of Dental Radiographs and Interpretation

Objectives

After completion of this chapter, the student will be able to:

▶ Summarize guidelines for prescribing the number, type and frequency of dental radiographs.

▶ Explain who benefits from dental radiographs, and list equipment and techniques used to limit radiation exposure.

▶ List uses for dental radiographs.

▶ Give examples of common dental anomalies, diseases, lesions and conditions that the dental professional may expect to find on dental radiographs.

▶ Summarize the importance of educating dental patients concerning dental radiographs.

▶ Define the terms *interpretation* and *diagnosis*.

▶ Define the roles of the dentist and dental hygienist in interpretation and diagnosis.

▶ Summarize the importance of radiographic interpretation.

▶ State the reasons for mounting dental radiographs.

▶ List and explain the proper equipment and viewing conditions necessary to interpret radiographs.

Key Words

Diagnosis
Film mounting
Film viewing
Interpretation

Dental radiographs are a necessary component of comprehensive patient care. In dentistry, radiographic examination is essential for diagnostic purposes. Radiographs enable the practitioner to identify many conditions that may otherwise go undetected; x-ray examinations enable the dental professional to see many conditions that are not apparent clinically. An intraoral examination, without the use of radiographs, is limited to what the practitioner can see clinically—the exposed surfaces of the teeth and the oral soft tissues. With the use of dental radiographs, the dental professional gains a great deal of information concerning the teeth and supporting bone. The purpose of this chapter is to review the importance of dental radiographs in comprehensive patient care, as well as the importance of interpretation and patient education concerning dental radiography.

THE IMPORTANCE OF DENTAL RADIOGRAPHS

The importance of dental radiographs as a diagnostic tool cannot be overemphasized. Radiographs play a critical role in diagnosis and patient care. The dental professional must have a working knowledge of the value and uses for dental radiographs.

How Many? How Often?

How many radiographs should be prescribed for a patient? How often should radiographic examinations take place? The decision to use radiographs in the diagnostic process is made by the dentist. The dentist's professional judgment is used to make decisions concerning the number, type and frequency of dental radiographs. Each patient's dental condition is different. Radiographs are prescribed for a patient based on the patient's individual needs. The decision to order radiographs is made after the patient's dental and medical histories are reviewed and a thorough clinical examination has been performed.

There is no set time limit between radiographic examinations. The decision concerning the frequency of radiographic examinations is also made based on the needs of the individual. The American Dental Association, through its Council on Dental Materials, Instruments and Equipment, has recommended that dental radiographic examinations never be routine or include a predetermined number of radiographs. The American Dental Association in conjunction with the Food and Drug Administration has adopted guidelines for prescribing the number, type and frequency of dental radiographs. These guidelines include a summary of recommendations that are intended to promote the safety and effectiveness of diagnostic radiology (Table 1–1).

Who Benefits from Dental Radiographs?

Dental radiographs are taken to benefit the patient. The primary benefit is the detection of disease. When radiographs are properly prescribed, exposed and processed, the benefit of detecting disease far outweighs the risk of small doses of x-ray exposure. Patients with questions concerning radiation safety need to be reassured that the prescribed radiographs are taken in an approved manner. The use of fast film, a collimated x-ray beam, proper filtration, a lead apron and thyroid collar, open-ended lead-lined cones and proper technique and processing all limit the amount of radiation received by the patient during a dental radiographic examination.

Through the proper use of radiographs, the dental professional can detect disease and ultimately benefit the patient by minimizing and preventing the possibility of toothaches or the need for surgical procedures. The dentist, by placing emphasis on the preventive aspect of radiography, can save the patient time and money while maintaining the patient in a state of oral health.

How Are Radiographs Used?

The uses for dental radiographs are many and varied. Radiographs can be utilized for the following:

- To detect diseases, lesions and conditions of teeth and bones that cannot be identified clinically.
- To confirm and/or classify suspected disease.
- To localize lesions or foreign objects.
- To provide information during dental treatment (e.g., endodontic treatment).
- To evaluate growth and development.
- To show changes secondary to caries, periodontal disease and trauma.
- To document the condition of a patient at a specific point in time.

TABLE 1–1. Guidelines for Prescribing Dental Radiographs

The recommendations in this chart are subject to clinical judgment and may not apply to every patient. They are to be used by dentists only after reviewing the patient's health history and completing a clinical examination. The recommendations do not need to be altered because of pregnancy.

Patient Category	Child — Primary Dentition *(prior to eruption of first permanent tooth)*	Child — Transitional Dentition *(following eruption of first permanent tooth)*	Adolescent — Permanent Dentition *(prior to eruption of third molars)*	Adult — Dentulous	Adult — Edentulous
New Patient* All new patients to assess dental diseases and growth and development	Posterior bite-wing examination if proximal surfaces of primary teeth cannot be visualized or probed	Individualized radiographic examination consisting of periapical/occlusal views and posterior bite-wings *or* panoramic examination and posterior bitewings	Individualized radiographic examination consisting of posterior bite-wings and selected periapicals. A full mouth intraoral radiographic examination is appropriate when the patient presents with clinical evidence of generalized dental disease or a history of extensive dental treatment.	*(see Adolescent)*	Full mouth intraoral radiographic examination *or* panoramic examination
Recall Patient* Clinical caries or high-risk factors for caries**	Posterior bite-wing examination at 6-month intervals *or* until no carious lesions are evident	*(see Primary Dentition)*	Posterior bite-wing examination at 6- to 12-month intervals *or* until no carious lesions are evident	Posterior bite-wing examination at 12- to 18-month intervals	Not applicable
No clinical caries and no high-risk factors for caries**	Posterior bite-wing examination at 12- to 24-month intervals if proximal surfaces of primary teeth cannot be visualized or probed	Posterior bite-wing examination at 12- to 24-month intervals	Posterior bite-wing examination at 18- to 36-month intervals	Posterior bite-wing examination at 24- to 36-month intervals	Not applicable
Periodontal disease or a history of periodontal treatment	Individualized radiographic examination consisting of selected periapical and/or bite-wing radiographs for areas where periodontal disease (other than nonspecific gingivitis) can be demonstrated clinically				Not applicable
Growth and development assessment	Usually not indicated	Individualized radiographic examination consisting of a periapical/occlusal *or* panoramic examination	Periapical *or* panoramic examination to assess developing third molars	Usually not indicated	Usually not indicated

* Clinical situations for which radiographs may be indicated include:

A. *Positive Historical findings*
1. Previous periodontal or endodontic therapy
2. History of pain or trauma
3. Familial history of dental anomalies
4. Postoperative evaluation of healing
5. Presence of implants

B. *Positive Clinical Signs/Symptoms*
1. Clinical evidence of periodontal disease
2. Large or deep restorations
3. Deep carious lesions
4. Malposed or clinically impacted teeth
5. Swelling
6. Evidence of facial trauma
7. Mobility of teeth
8. Fistula or sinus tract infection
9. Clinically suspected sinus pathology
10. Growth abnormalities
11. Oral involvement in known or suspected systemic disease
12. Positive neurologic findings in the head and neck
13. Evidence of foreign objects
14. Pain and/or dysfunction of the temporomandibular joint
15. Facial asymmetry
16. Abutment teeth for fixed or removable partial prosthesis
17. Unexplained bleeding
18. Unexplained sensitivity of teeth
19. Unusual eruption, spacing or migration of teeth
20. Unusual tooth morphology; calcification or color
21. Missing teeth with unknown reason

** Patients at high risk for caries may demonstrate any of the following:
1. High level of caries experience
2. History of recurrent caries
3. Existing restoration of poor quality
4. Poor oral hygiene
5. Inadequate fluoride exposure
6. Prolonged nursing (bottle or breast)
7. Diet with high sucrose frequency
8. Poor family dental health
9. Developmental enamel defects
10. Developmental disability
11. Xerostomia
12. Genetic abnormality of teeth
13. Many multisurface restorations
14. Chemo/radiation therapy

The recommendations contained in this table have been developed by an expert panel comprised of representatives from the Academy of General Dentistry, American Academy of Dental Radiology, American Academy of Oral Medicine, American Academy of Pediatric Dentistry, American Academy of Periodontology and the American Dental Association under the sponsorship of the Food and Drug Administration (FDA). This chart has been reproduced and distributed to the dental community by Eastman Kodak Company in cooperation with the FDA. (Reprinted courtesy of Eastman Kodak Company.)

The dental professional must be able to communicate information concerning the value and use of radiographs to the dental patient. Many patients do not understand the importance of dental radiographs. It is the responsibility of the dental professional to emphasize the fact that many dental diseases and conditions produce no clinical signs or symptoms and are typically discovered *only* through the use of dental radiographs. One of the most important uses for dental radiographs is *detection*. Radiographs allow the practitioner to detect lesions, diseases and conditions of the teeth and bones that cannot be identified clinically. Patients need to understand that without a radiographic examination, many diseases, lesions and conditions of the jaws may go undetected.

The patient must be made aware of the benefits of early diagnosis and treatment. When clinically undetectable conditions exist, early detection and diagnosis through the use of dental radiographs benefits the patient. Early treatment usually results in less discomfort for the patient and prevents further destruction of affected structures and unnecessary loss of teeth. In cases of malignant lesions, early detection and diagnosis through the use of dental radiographs often affect the overall prognosis.

Dental radiographs are not only used for detection but also for confirming suspected diseases and assisting in the localization of lesions and foreign objects. Radiographs provide essential information during routine dental treatment; for example, the dentist depends on radiographs during root canal procedures. Dental radiographs can be used to examine the state of teeth and bone in the evaluation of growth and development. Dental radiographs are indispensable in showing changes secondary to trauma, caries and periodontal disease.

Dental radiographs are an essential component of the patient record. A radiograph contains an incredible amount of information, far more than a written record. An initial radiographic examination provides baseline information concerning the patient. Each radiograph serves to document the condition of a patient during a certain point in time. Radiographs taken at a later date can be compared to those taken earlier. Films can be compared for changes from treatment, trauma or disease.

What Can Be Found on a Radiograph?

Numerous conditions of the jaws produce no clinical signs or symptoms and can *only* can be detected radiographically. Some of the more common diseases, lesions and conditions that the dental professional may expect to find on dental radiographs include developing permanent teeth, missing and supernumerary teeth, impacted teeth, dental caries, recurrent caries, periodontal disease, dilacerated roots, retained roots and periapical lesions. Example radiographs can be used to educate the dental patient concerning some of these common conditions that are only detected through the use of dental radiographs.

Developing Permanent Teeth

Developing permanent teeth cannot be monitored clinically. The dental radiograph can be used to reveal the presence or absence of developing teeth. In cases of delayed eruption, a radiograph can be used to verify the presence of a permanent tooth. Figure 1–1 illustrates an example of an erupting permanent mandibular premolar.

Missing Teeth

Missing teeth can be verified using a dental radiograph. Figure 1–2 illustrates a case of a missing premolar.

Missing teeth may result in occlusion problems from drifting or tipping. Orthodontic evaluation and/or treatment may be necessary. When missing teeth are discovered early through the use of dental radiographs, steps can be implemented to prevent occlusion problems. Patients with multiple missing teeth should be evaluated for the presence of syndromes such as hereditary ectodermal dysplasia, Böök's syndrome and Rieger's syndrome.

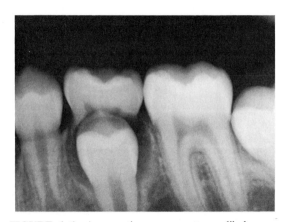

FIGURE 1–1. An erupting permanent mandibular premolar.

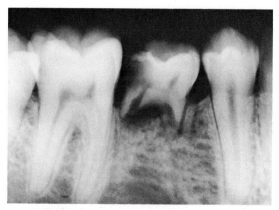

FIGURE 1–2. A missing mandibular premolar.

Supernumerary Teeth

Supernumerary or extra teeth may also be identified on a dental radiograph. Figure 1–3 is an example of two supernumerary teeth, one erupted and one impacted. Most supernumerary teeth are discovered as incidental radiographic findings. Erupted supernumerary teeth may cause crowding, malpositioning of adjacent teeth or noneruption of normal teeth. Nonerupted supernumerary teeth have the potential for dentigerous cyst formation. For this reason, nonerupted supernumerary teeth should be extracted. Patients with multiple supernumerary teeth should be evaluated for cleidocranial dysplasia and Gardner's syndrome.

Impacted Teeth

Impacted teeth are one of the most common developmental defects in humans. Any tooth may be impacted; the most common impacted teeth include the maxillary and mandibular third molars, maxillary cuspids, maxillary and mandibular premolars and supernumerary teeth. Impacted teeth are identified radiographically.

Figure 1–4 illustrates an example of an impacted third molar. Impacted teeth should be removed surgically to prevent odontogenic cyst formation, damage of adjacent teeth and bone resorption resulting in susceptibility to fractures.

Dental Caries

While a number of carious lesions can be detected clinically, a great percentage of them cannot. With such lesions, a radiograph is necessary. The bite-wing radiograph is indispensable in the detection of interproximal carious lesions.

Figure 1–5 illustrates a severe carious lesion on the distal of tooth #19 and an advanced carious lesion on the mesial of tooth #18. Dental caries, if left untreated, can result in the destruction of a large amount of tooth structure and pulpal necrosis. Early detection and treatment of carious lesions can prevent further damage to tooth structure.

Recurrent Caries

Decay may recur under the margins of existing restorations. Recurrent caries may or may not be evident clinically. A dental radiograph helps to detect and diagnose recurrent caries. Figure 1–6 illustrates an example of recurrent decay located under the amalgam restoration on tooth #30. Recurrent dental caries, if left untreated, results in tooth destruction and pulpal necrosis. Early detection of recurrent carious lesions through the use of dental radiographs can prevent further damage to tooth structure.

Periodontal Disease

Periodontal disease cannot be diagnosed without dental radiographs. The diagnosis of periodontal disease must include a combination of

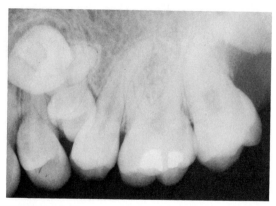

FIGURE 1–3. Two supernumerary teeth, one erupted and one impacted.

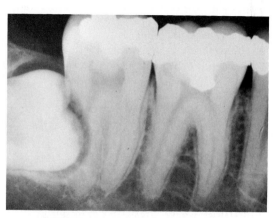

FIGURE 1–4. An impacted third molar.

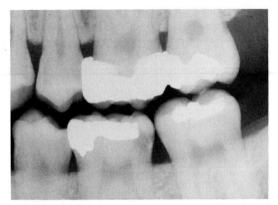

FIGURE 1–5. Dental caries on the distal surface of tooth #19 and the mesial surface of tooth #18.

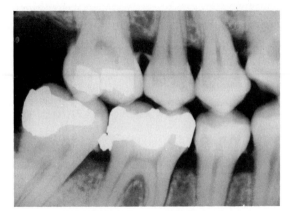

FIGURE 1–7. Interproximal calculus.

radiographs and a thorough clinical exam. Dental radiographs serve to identify predisposing factors (e.g., calculus or faulty restorations), detect bony or crestal changes and furcation involvements, approximate the amount and location of bone loss and aid in the evaluation and prognosis of the affected teeth. Dental radiographs also provide baseline information concerning the periodontium. The baseline information can then be used as a pretreatment reference source.

Figure 1–7 illustrates an example of interproximal calculus and associated bone loss seen with periodontal disease.

Dilacerated Roots

Tooth root morphology is not apparent clinically. Many teeth exhibit root dilaceration or the abnormal bending or curvature of a root. The dental radiograph allows the dental professional to view both the crown and roots of the tooth.

Figure 1–8 illustrates an example of root dilaceration. Teeth that exhibit dilacerated roots

are often difficult to extract or treat endodontically. The dental radiograph provides the practitioner with essential information concerning root dilacerations.

Retained Roots

Root tips or fragments are sometimes left behind following a difficult tooth extraction. Retained roots are usually asymptomatic and are often only discovered during radiographic examination. Figure 1–9 illustrates an example of a retained deciduous root tip between teeth #29 and #30. Usually, retained root fragments do not require removal. However, root fragments should be periodically reevaluated with the use of dental radiographs.

Periapical Lesions

Periapical lesions may also be discovered during the radiographic examination. A number of lesions may appear in the periapical regions. The

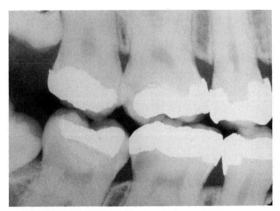

FIGURE 1–6. Recurrent decay on tooth #30.

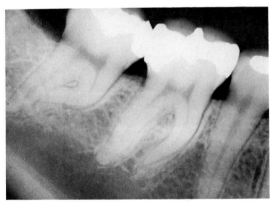

FIGURE 1–8. Root dilaceration.

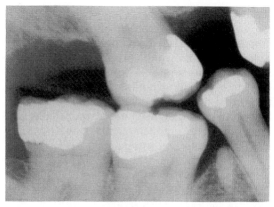

FIGURE 1–9. Retained deciduous root tip.

most common radiographic appearance of a periapical lesion is the radiolucency seen at the tooth apex.

Figure 1–10 illustrates an example of a radiolucency at the apex of tooth #19. A diagnosis of a periapical cyst, granuloma or abscess cannot be made based on the radiographic findings alone. Histologic examination of the periapical tissue is necessary to make the definitive diagnosis.

Other Lesions

Numerous dental anomalies, cysts, tumors and diseases affect the jaws. Lesions may persist for years before signs or symptoms develop. The dental radiographic examination plays a vital role in the detection and diagnosis of such lesions. Lesions identified early cause less destruction and are more easily treated. The importance of early detection and diagnosis cannot be overstated.

Why Patient Education?

Educating patients about the value of dental radiography is often overlooked by dental professionals. As previously mentioned, many patients do not understand the importance of dental radiographs. Many patients fear the use of radiation, and others believe that dental radiographs are a way for the dentist to make money. In order to address such patient fears and misconceptions, the dental professional must be prepared to educate the patient regarding the value of dental radiographs.

The dental professional must be able to explain exactly how dental radiographs are used and how they benefit the patient. In addition, the dental professional must be able to provide examples of common conditions and lesions detected by dental radiographs.

Patient education can take place in a variety of ways. One effective way to communicate information is an oral presentation. Oral explanations or presentations along with sample radiographs can be used to discuss the importance of dental radiographs (Fig. 1–11). Through the use of radiographs, the dental professional can introduce a visual component to the educational process. Visual aids enhance patient comprehension. The dental professional can put together a series of radiographs that illustrate typical normal and abnormal dental conditions (see Figs. 1–1 through 1–10). A prepared oral presentation with visual aids allows patients to develop a greater confidence in the expertise of the dental professional. Educational presentations prepared in advance enhance the dental professional's appearance of being organized and competent.

Printed information about dental radiographs

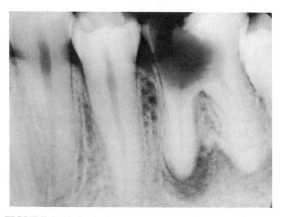

FIGURE 1–10. Periapical radiolucency at the apex of tooth #19.

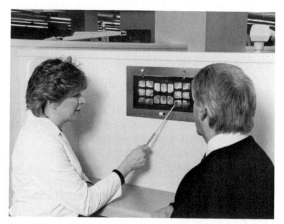

FIGURE 1–11. The dental hygienist can communicate important information concerning dental radiographs during an informal oral presentation.

is also helpful. Brochures can be placed in the reception area of the dental office or distributed to patients before the radiographic examination. "Dental X-Rays: Their Purpose and Use," a pamphlet that can be obtained from the American Dental Association, is one example of the printed literature that is available. This pamphlet, in very basic terms, explains what x-rays do and how dental radiographs benefit the patient. The use of printed literature can be used in conjunction with an oral presentation or can be used to provide a basis for a question-and-answer discussion about the importance of dental radiographs.

Currently, many dental offices do not educate their patients concerning the importance of dental radiographs. Often, the patient is simply told that dental x-rays are required by the dentist and very little information or additional explanation is given. Educating patients should not be limited to demonstrations on flossing and brushing; it must also include discussing the value of dental radiographs and emphasizing their preventive aspect. Proper patient education results in decreased fears of x-ray exposure and increased cooperation and motivation for regular dental visits.

THE IMPORTANCE OF RADIOGRAPHIC INTERPRETATION

Radiographic interpretation is of paramount importance to the dental professional. The ability to evaluate and recognize what is revealed by a radiograph enables the dental professional to play a vital role in the detection of diseases, lesions and conditions of the teeth and jaws that cannot be identified clinically.

Interpretation Versus Diagnosis

Radiographic interpretation can be defined as the ability to read what is revealed by a radiograph. In the dental setting, the terms **interpretation** and **diagnosis** are often confused; it is important to note that these terms have very different meanings. An *interpretation* is an explanation of what is viewed on a radiograph. Both the dentist and dental hygienist are trained to interpret radiographs. However, only the dentist is specifically trained to render a diagnosis. The term *diagnosis* is derived from two Greek words: *dia* "through" and *gnosis*

"knowledge". *Diagnosis* can be defined as "to know apart" or "to distinguish." In dentistry, a *diagnosis* is made by the dentist after a thorough review, evaluation and correlation of the following: the medicodental history, clinical examination, radiographic examination and clinical and laboratory tests. The final interpretation of radiographs and diagnosis are responsibilities of the dentist. The dental hygienist is restricted, by law, from rendering a diagnosis.

Interpretation and the Dental Hygienist

If the dentist is responsible for the final interpretation of radiographs and diagnosis, what then is the role of the dental hygienist? The dental hygienist can play an important role in the preliminary interpretation of dental radiographs. In order to play such a role, the dental hygienist must be confident in the identification and recognition of normal anatomic landmarks, common variations of normal anatomy, periodontal disease, dental caries, restorative materials, common lesions, dental anomalies and traumatic injuries to bone. The dental hygienist who prepares a preliminary interpretation can present the findings to the dentist along with the clinical findings obtained during patient examination. As an additional pair of eyes viewing the films, the dental hygienist can direct the dentist's attention to areas of question or concern. Such a preliminary interpretation results in a more efficient use of time for both the dentist and dental hygienist.

Interpretation and Use of Radiographs

Radiographs contain a wealth of information. *All* radiographs must be reviewed and interpreted. Films that are not interpreted are like books that go unread—the information is present but has yet to be discovered. All too often, radiographs are taken at the end of a dental appointment and reviewed in a cursory manner without the patient present. In many instances, radiographs are reviewed by dentists and then hidden away in the patient folder.

It is essential to remember that radiographs are taken to benefit the patient. Therefore, radiographs should be taken at the beginning of the dental appointment, utilized for diagnostic and educational purposes at the initial appointment and utilized at subsequent appointments as well. Dental radiographs should be interpreted by the dental professional with the patient present. If any suspicious or questionable areas are viewed on the films, the patient can be examined to obtain additional information or to confirm what is suspected radiographically. If the dental professional interprets radiographs without the patient present, much needed clinical information is lacking.

Interpretation and Patient Education

Interpretation of patient radiographs can be used as an educational tool in the dental office. Besides providing a preliminary interpretation of dental radiographs, the dental hygienist can educate the patient by identifying and discussing what can normally be found on a dental radiograph. Then the dentist can focus on specific problems or areas of concern identified or treatment planning. This example of how the dentist and dental hygienist can work together using radiographic interpretation is one way in which dental professionals can educate patients concerning the importance and use of dental radiographs.

Preparation for Interpretation

Dental radiographs must be prepared for interpretation. Films must be mounted prior to viewing. Proper film mounting and viewing techniques are essential in the interpretation of dental radiographs.

Film Mounting

What Is a Film Mount?
A **film mount** is a cardboard or plastic holder that is used to arrange dental radiographs in anatomic order. Anatomic order refers to how the teeth are arranged within the dental arches. Mounted films are invaluable to the dental professional; a series of mounted radiographs can be viewed more efficiently than individual films, one by one. The windows or frames in a film mount are available in many sizes and combinations and can accommodate any number of films from a full series to a set of bite-wings to one intraoral film (Fig. 1–12).

Why Use a Film Mount?
The use of a film mount is suggested for the following reasons:

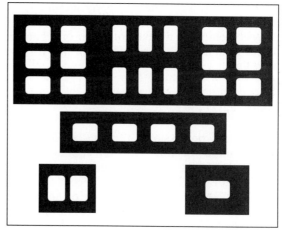

FIGURE 1–12. A variety of film mounts are available in many sizes and film combinations.

- Mounted radiographs are easier to view and interpret.
- Film mounts aid in eliminating the confusion of the patient's right and left.
- Mounted radiographs are easily filed in patient folders and are readily accessible for interpretation.
- Film mounts decrease handling of individual films and prevent fingerprint marks and scratches.
- Film mounts mask illumination immediately adjacent to individual radiographs and aid in interpretation.

Who Mounts Films?
Any trained dental professional (dentist, dental hygienist or dental assistant) with a knowledge of normal radiographic landmarks is qualified to mount dental radiographs.

What Information Is Placed on a Film Mount?
All film mounts must be labeled. Radiographs can be easily identified when the film mount has been clearly and legibly labeled with the following information:

- Patient's full name.
- Date of exposure.
- Dentist's name.
- Radiographer's name.

When and Where Are Films Mounted?
Radiographs should be mounted immediately after processing. Films should be mounted in an area designated for film mounting. This area should consist of a clean, dry, light-colored work surface in front of an illuminator or viewbox.

After films have been properly mounted, labeled, viewed and interpreted, they should always be placed in the patient folder or record in order to eliminate the possibility of film loss or mix-up.

Film Viewing

The dental professional requires an adequate light source for **film viewing,** subdued room lighting and magnification in order to interpret dental radiographs.

Light Source. A light source or an illuminator (viewbox) is required to accurately view radiographs and assist in interpretation of images. The viewing area of the illuminator should be large enough to accommodate a variety of mounted films as well as unmounted extraoral films. The illumination should be of uniform intensity and evenly diffused. If the screen of the illuminator is not completely covered by the mounted radiographs, the harsh light around the mounted films should be masked in order to reduce glare and intensify the detail and contrast of the radiographic images (Fig. 1–13).

Room Lighting. The dental professional who is interpreting radiographs must concentrate and pay close attention to detail. An area free of distractions with subdued room lighting is recommended for interpretation of dental radiographs.

Magnification. The use of a pocket-sized magnifying glass is useful to the dental professional in radiographic interpretation. Magnification aids the viewer in evaluating slight changes in density and contrast present in radiographic images (Fig. 1–14).

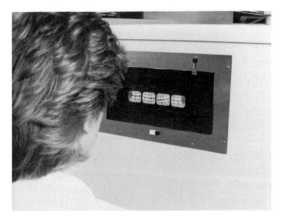

FIGURE 1–13. Extraneous light should be masked in order to reduce glare and intensify the contrast of the radiographic image.

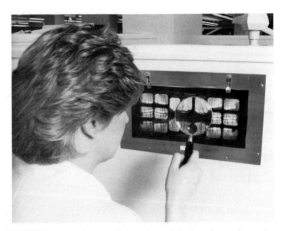

FIGURE 1–14. A magnifying glass aids the viewer in evaluation of subtle changes in density and contrast.

SUMMARY

In dentistry, the use of radiographs is essential for diagnostic purposes. The dental professional must be familiar with the guidelines for prescribing the number, type and frequency of dental radiographs. Radiographs must be prescribed for a patient based on that patient's individual needs. Radiographic examinations should *never* be routine or include a predetermined number of radiographs.

The dental professional must remember that radiographs are taken to benefit the patient. The main benefit is disease detection. Through the use of radiographs, the dental professional can detect disease and prevent the possibility of tooth loss or the need for surgery. Without them, the patient may needlessly experience pain, discomfort, loss of function or poor esthetics. Also, conditions that are allowed to worsen require more time and money.

The dental professional must have a thorough knowledge concerning the value and uses for dental radiographs. Because radiographs play a critical role in diagnosis and patient care, the dental professional must be able to educate the patient concerning the importance of dental radiographs. Dental health education is one of the greatest services the dental professional can provide to the dental patient. Dental education should not only include oral health and restorative dentistry but also the importance of radiographs as well.

Radiographic interpretation, or the ability to read what is revealed by a radiograph, is an important component of patient care. The dental hygienist is restricted by law from making diagnoses but can facilitate patient care by presenting a preliminary radiographic interpretation.

The dental hygienist and dentist can work together to educate patients about the importance and use of dental radiographs.

Radiographs should be taken at the beginning of the appointment and interpreted with the patient in the chair. Radiographs should be properly mounted and labeled before interpretation. An illuminator, subdued room lighting and a magnifying glass are necessary for optimum interpretation.

Bibliography

Dental X-rays: Their Purpose and Use. Chicago: American Dental Association, 1982.

Council on Dental Materials, Instruments and Equipment: Recommendations in radiographic practices: an update 1988. JADA 1989; 118:115–17.

Guidelines for Prescribing Dental Radiographs. Rochester, NY: Eastman Kodak, 1988.

Barr JH and Stephens RG: The diagnostic context of radiographic findings. *In* Dental Radiology: Pertinent Basic Concepts and Their Applications in Clinical Practice, pp 350–75. Philadelphia: WB Saunders, 1980.

DeLyre WR and Johnson ON: Patient education. *In* Essentials of Dental Radiography for Dental Assistants and Hygienists, 4th ed., pp 375–83. Norwalk, CT: Appleton and Lange, 1990.

Goaz PW and White SC. Principles of radiographic interpretation. *In* Oral Radiology and Principles of Interpretation, 2d ed., pp 161–73. St. Louis: CV Mosby, 1987.

Langland OE, Sippy FH and Langlais RP: Principles of interpretation of pathologic conditions. *In* Textbook of Dental Radiography, 2d ed., pp 367–79. Springfield, IL: Charles C Thomas, 1984.

Manson-Hing LR: Patient relations. *In* Fundamentals of Dental Radiography, 3d ed., pp 221–229. Philadelphia: Lea and Febiger, 1990.

Manson-Hing LR: Interpretation and value of radiographs. *In* Fundamentals of Dental Radiography, 3d ed., pp 201–220. Philadelphia: Lea and Febiger, 1990.

QUIZ QUESTIONS

1. Which of the following statements are true?

   (1) The decision to use radiographs in the diagnostic process is made by the dentist.
   (2) Every patient's dental condition is different.
   (3) Dental radiographic examinations should be routine and consist of a predetermined number of films.

   a. 1 and 2
   b. 1 and 3
   c. 2 and 3
   d. all of the above

2. List four ways to limit the amount of radiation received by the patient during a radiographic exam.

   (1) _____
   (2) _____
   (3) _____
   (4) _____

3. Which of the following is the most important use for dental radiographs?

   a. to evaluate growth and development
   b. detection
   c. to localize lesions or foreign objects
   d. to provide information during dental treatment

4. Which of the following dental conditions requires the use of radiographs for identification or detection?

   (1) interproximal dental caries
   (2) dilacerated roots
   (3) impacted teeth
   (4) periapical lesions

   a. 1, 2, and 3
   b. 1, 2, and 4
   c. 2, 3, and 4
   d. all of the above

5. Dental radiographs are taken to benefit the patient.

   _____ true
   _____ false

6. Matching

   ____ interpretation   **a.** responsible for the final interpretation of radiographs
   ____ diagnosis   **b.** to know apart or distinguish
   ____ dentist   **c.** an explanation of what is viewed on a radiograph
   ____ dental hygienist   **d.** can provide a preliminary interpretation and present findings

7. Which of the following is *false* concerning film mounting?

   a. mounted radiographs are easier to view
   b. film mounts decrease the chance of fingerprints on films
   c. unmounted films can be interpreted as easily as mounted films
   d. film mounts mask illumination around individual films

8. Name three essential conditions for viewing films.

   (1) _____

   (2) _____

   (3) _____

9. *Case Study Question:* A 24-year-old male law student presents to a local dental office for a dental prophylaxis. The patient's last dental appointment was approximately 3½ years ago. The patient, when questioned about his dental x-ray history, states that he is opposed to "excess" exposure to radiation, especially in the absence of tooth pain or problems. As a dental hygienist, what will you tell this patient in order to educate him concerning the importance of dental radiographs?

CHAPTER TWO

Descriptive Terminology

Objectives

After completion of this chapter, the student will be able to:

▶ Identify the categories of information that should be documented for all lesions viewed radiographically.

▶ Define "descriptive terminology" and describe why it should be used by the dental professional.

▶ Define the terms *radiograph, x-ray, radiolucent* and *radiopaque.*

▶ Differentiate between the terms *radiograph* and *x-ray.*

▶ Differentiate between the terms *radiolucent* and *radiopaque.*

▶ Define the terms *unilocular* and *multilocular.*

▶ Define the terms *periapical, inter-radicular, edentulous zone, pericoronal* and *alveolar bone loss.*

▶ Identify radiolucent lesions on a radiograph in terms of appearance, location and size.

▶ Define the terms *focal opacity, target lesion, multifocal confluent, irregular/ill-defined, ground glass, mixed lucent-opaque* and *soft tissue opacity.*

▶ Identify radiopaque lesions on a radiograph in terms of appearance, location and size.

Key Words

Alveolar bone loss	Pericoronal
Edentulous zone	Radiograph
Focal opacity	Radiolucent
Ground glass	Radiopaque
Inter-radicular	Soft tissue opacity
Irregular, expansile	Target lesion
Mixed lucent-opaque	Unilocular corticated
Multifocal confluent	Unilocular noncorticated
Multilocular	X-ray
Periapical	

Interpretation, as defined in Chapter 1, is the ability to read what is revealed by a radiograph. In order to interpret dental radiographs, the dental professional must be able to accurately and succinctly describe what is observed. A working knowledge of descriptive terminology is important for communication and documentation and is essential in radiographic interpretation.

DESCRIPTIVE TERMINOLOGY

What Is Descriptive Terminology?

In dental radiography, a number of terms can be used to describe the appearance, location and size of a lesion. This information should be documented for *all* lesions viewed radiographically.

Why Use Descriptive Terminology?

Descriptive terminology allows dental professionals to intelligently describe and discuss what is seen on a dental radiograph and to communicate using a common language. Communication among dental professionals about radiographic findings takes place each time a patient case is discussed or when a patient is referred to a specialist for evaluation. The use of descriptive terminology eliminates the chance for miscommunication among dental professionals.

Descriptive terminology also allows the dental professional to document what is seen on a radiograph in the patient record in terms of appearance, location and size. Documentation of what is viewed on dental radiographs is essential for legal purposes. A written description of what is viewed on a radiograph indicates that the dental professional interpreted the x-ray film. If no notation of interpretation is included in the patient record, there is no documentation that the films were reviewed.

Descriptive Terminology Versus Diagnosis

Is describing a lesion the same as making a diagnosis? Descriptive terminology allows the dental hygienist to describe what is seen on a radiograph *without* implying a diagnosis. It is important to note that it is extremely difficult, if not impossible, to diagnose from a radiograph alone. Correlation and review of additional information, including the patient's medical and dental history, clinical findings, signs and symptoms, laboratory tests and biopsy results, are necessary in order for the dentist to make a definitive diagnosis.

Review of Basic Terms

The use of descriptive terminology requires that the dental professional has a basic understanding of four general terms: *radiograph, x-ray, radiolucent,* and *radiopaque*.

Radiograph Versus X-Ray

Although the terms *radiograph* and *x-ray* are often used interchangeably by the dental professional it is important to note that these two terms have very distinct and different meanings.

A **radiograph** is an image that is produced on photosensitive film by exposing the film to x-rays and then processing the film so that a negative is produced. A radiograph may also be called x-ray film, radiogram, roentgenogram or roentgenograph.

The terms *radiograph* and *x-ray* are *not* synonymous. A radiograph refers to the actual *film* exposed, and an x-ray refers to the *beam of energy,* or radiation. Therefore, the dental professional should not refer to a radiograph as an x-ray but rather an x-ray film.

An **x-ray,** or **roentgen ray,** is a beam of energy that has the power to penetrate substances and to record shadow images on photographic film.

Radiolucent Versus Radiopaque

The terms *radiolucent* and *radiopaque* are used to describe the appearance of all structures seen on a radiograph. A radiograph appears radiolucent (black or dark) where the tissues are soft or thin and radiopaque (white or light) where the tissues are thick or hard. Most structures radiographed do not exhibit uniform thicknesses and therefore appear gray instead of black or white.

Radiolucent refers to that portion of a processed radiograph that is dark or black. Radiolucent structures lack density and permit the passage of the x-ray beam with little or no resistance.

Dental caries appears radiolucent (Fig. 2–1) because the area of tooth with caries is less

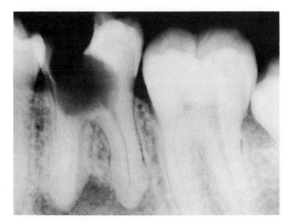

FIGURE 2–1. Dental caries appears radiolucent on a radiograph.

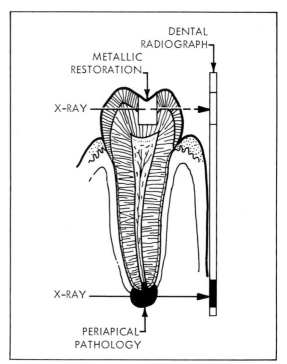

FIGURE 2–2. This diagram shows variations of x-ray absorption in a tooth with an amalgam restoration and periapical lesion. The amalgam restoration *absorbs* the x-ray beam. The x-ray beam does not reach the film surface and a white or *radiopaque* area results. The lesion at the apex of the tooth lacks density and is *easily penetrated* by the x-ray beam. The beam reaches the film and results in a dark or *radiolucent* area. (Modified from Langland OE, Sippy FH, and Langlais RP: Textbook of Dental Radiography, 2d ed. Springfield, IL: Charles C Thomas, 1984.)

dense than surrounding structures and therefore readily permits the passage of the x-ray beam. Consequently, most of the energy of the x-ray beam freely passes through the area of caries to the recording surface of the radiograph resulting in a dark or radiolucent area on the film (Fig. 2–2). Other radiolucent structures include airspaces, soft tissues, dental pulp and the periodontal ligament space.

Radiopaque refers to that portion of a processed radiograph that appears light or white. Radiopaque structures are dense and absorb or resist the passage of the x-ray beam.

A metallic restoration appears radiopaque (Fig. 2–3) because it is very dense and absorbs the radiation. As a result, very little, if any, radiation reaches the surface of the film and results in a white or radiopaque area on the film (see Fig. 2–2). Examples of other radiopaque structures include enamel, dentin and bone.

Terms Used to Describe Radiolucent Lesions

A number of terms can be used to describe lesions found on radiographs. A lesion that appears radiolucent permits the passage of the x-ray beam and represents a destruction of bone or a space-occupying entity within the bones of the jaws. Radiolucent lesions may be described in terms of appearance, location and size.

Appearance

The appearance of most radiolucent lesions can be classified as either unilocular or multilocular. Other radiolucent classifications include a moth-eaten pattern, a multifocal pattern or a widened periodontal ligament space. Examples of radiolucent lesions in each of these categories can be found listed in Table 2–1.

Unilocular Radiolucent Lesions. The term *unilocular* is derived from two Latin words, *uni* ("one") and *loculus* ("small space" or "compartment"). Unilocular refers to a radiolucent lesion that exhibits one compartment. Unilocular lesions tend to be small and nonexpansile. Unilocular lesions have borders that

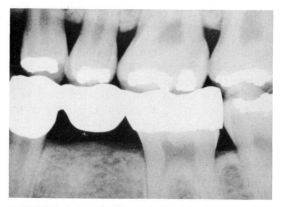

FIGURE 2–3. A gold bridge appears radiopaque on a radiograph.

TABLE 2–1. Radiolucent Lesions of the Jaws

Unilocular Radiolucencies	Moth-Eaten Radiolucencies
Periapical cyst	Osteomyelitis
Periapical granuloma	Metastatic carcinoma†
Periapical abscess	Osteosarcoma*†
Periapical cemental dysplasia*†	Chondrosarcoma*†
	Ewing's sarcoma
Incisive canal cyst	Lymphoma
Traumatic bone cyst	Burkitt's lymphoma
Residual bone cyst	Fibrosarcoma
Lateral periodontal cyst	Multiple myeloma*
Odontogenic keratocyst*	
Primordial cyst	**Widened Periodontal Ligament Space**
Osteoporotic bone marrow defect	
	Scleroderma
Dentigerous cyst	Osteosarcoma*
Static bone cyst	Periodontal inflammation
Ameloblastoma*	Endodontic inflammation
Adenomatoid odontogenic tumor†	
Calcifying epithelial odontogenic tumor*†	
Ameloblastic fibroma*	
Central giant cell granuloma*	

Multilocular Radiolucencies	Multifocal Radiolucencies
Odontogenic keratocyst*	Basal cell nevus syndrome
Ameloblastoma*	Histiocytosis X
Central giant cell granuloma	Multiple myeloma*
Botryoid odontogenic cyst	Cherubism†
Aneursymal bone cyst	Periapical cemental dysplasia*†
Cherubism*	
Hyperparathyroidism	
Myxoma	
Central neurogenic neoplasms	
Ameloblastic fibroma*	
Calcifying epithelial odontogenic tumor*†	

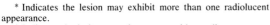

* Indicates the lesion may exhibit more than one radiolucent appearance.

† Indicates the lesion may also appear with a radiopaque component.

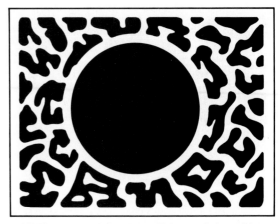

FIGURE 2–4. A unilocular radiolucent lesion with corticated borders. (Modified from Eversole LR: Clinical Outline of Oral Pathology: Diagnosis and Treatment, 2d ed. Philadephia: Lea and Febiger, 1984.)

may appear corticated or noncorticated on the radiograph.

Unilocular Lesion, Corticated Borders. The term *corticated* comes from the Latin *cortex* ("an outer layer") and refers to the outer layer or border of a radiolucent lesion. A unilocular radiolucent lesion with corticated borders exhibits a thin, well-demarcated radiopaque rim of bone at the periphery (Fig. 2–4). A unilocular lesion with corticated borders is usually indicative of a benign slow-growing process.

Unilocular Lesion, Noncorticated Borders. A unilocular lesion with noncorticated borders does *not* exhibit a thin radiopaque rim of bone at the periphery (Fig. 2–5). Instead, the periphery of a unilocular, noncorticated lesion appears fuzzy or ill-defined. Radiolucencies

with ill-defined or irregular margins may represent either a benign or malignant process.

Multilocular Radiolucent Lesions. The term *multilocular* refers to a lesion which exhibits multiple radiolucent compartments (Fig. 2–6). A lesion with multiple compartments is larger than a lesion with one compartment; therefore, by definition, a multilocular lesion is larger than a unilocular lesion. Multilocular lesions typically exhibit well-defined, corticated margins. Multilocular radiolucent lesions are frequently expansile and tend to displace the buccal and/or lingual plates of bone.

Multilocular lesions are typically benign lesions with aggressive growth potential. As a general rule, most multilocular lesions represent a reactive or neoplastic process. The odontogenic keratocyst, ameloblastoma and the central

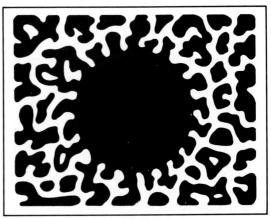

FIGURE 2–5. A unilocular radiolucent lesion with noncorticated borders. (Modified from Eversole LR: Clinical Outline of Oral Pathology: Diagnosis and Treatment, 2d ed. Philadephia: Lea and Febiger, 1984.)

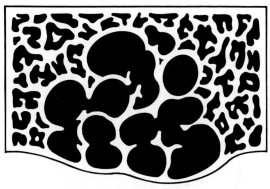

FIGURE 2–6. A multilocular radiolucent lesion. (Modified from Eversole LR: Clinical Outline of Oral Pathology: Diagnosis and Treatment, 2d ed. Philadelphia: Lea and Febiger, 1984.)

TABLE 2–2. Locations of Radiolucent Lesions

Periapical Radiolucencies	Pericoronal Radiolucencies
Periapical cyst	Dentigerous cyst
Periapical granuloma	Odontogenic keratocyst*
Periapical abscess	Ameloblastoma*
Periapical cemental	Adenomatoid odontogenic
dysplasia†	tumor†
Incisive canal cyst	Calcifying epithelial
Traumatic bone cyst*	odontogenic tumor†
Residual cyst*	
Odontogenic keratocyst*	**Alveolar Bone Loss**
Central giant cell	
granuloma	Periodontitis
	Histiocytosis X
Inter-radicular	Cyclic neutropenia
Radiolucencies	Leukemia
Lateral periodontal cyst	**No Specific Location**
Residual cyst*	
Odontogenic keratocyst*	Multiple myeloma
Primordial cyst*	Cherubism
Traumatic bone cyst*	Myxoma
Botryoid odontogenic cyst	Osteosarcoma†
	Osteomyelitis
Edentulous zone	Metastatic carcinoma†
	Chondrosarcoma†
Periapical cyst‡	Ewing's sarcoma
Periapical granuloma‡	Lymphoma
Periapical abscess‡	Burkitt's lymphoma
Periapical cemental	Fibrosarcoma
dysplasia*†‡	Multiple myeloma
Incisive canal cyst‡	Osteoporotic bone marrow
Residual cyst‡	defect
Odontogenic keratocyst*	Ameloblastic fibroma
Central giant cell	Aneurysmal bone cyst
granuloma*	Hyperparathyroidism
Primordial cyst*	
Ameloblastoma*	
Calcifying epithelial	
odontogenic tumor*†	
Static bone cyst	

* Indicates the lesion may exhibit more than one location.
† Indicates the lesion may also appear with a radiopaque component.
‡ Indicates this location is possible, postextraction of a related tooth.

giant cell granuloma are examples of multi-locular radiolucencies viewed on radiographs.

Location

In addition to appearance, radiolucent lesions can also be described in terms of location. The location of a lesion is important for communication and documentation purposes. A radiolucent lesion may appear in the periapical, inter-radicular, edentulous or pericoronal location. A radiolucent lesion may also appear as alveolar bone loss. Examples of radiolucent lesions and their most likely locations can be found in Table 2–2.

Periapical Location. The term *periapical* refers to a lesion located around the apex of a tooth (Fig. 2–7). It is derived from the Greek word *peri* ("around") and the Latin word *apex*, meaning the terminal end of a tooth root. An example of a common periapical radiolucency is a periapical cyst seen secondary to pulpal necrosis.

Inter-radicular Location. The term *inter-radicular* refers to a lesion located between the roots of adjacent teeth (Fig. 2–8). *Inter* is Latin for "between," and "radicular" means pertaining to a root. An example of a radiolucent lesion that would be expected to be found in the inter-radicular location is the lateral periodontal cyst.

Edentulous Zone. The term *edentulous zone* refers to a lesion located in an area without teeth (Fig. 2–9). (*Edentulous* means "without teeth.") A variety of radiolucent lesions may occur in the edentulous zone.

Pericoronal Location. The term *pericoronal* refers to a radiolucent lesion located around the crown of an impacted tooth (Fig. 2–10). (*Peri* is Greek for "around," and *corona* is Latin for "crown.") A dentigerous cyst is an example of a radiolucent lesion seen in the pericoronal location.

Alveolar Bone Loss. The term *alveolar bone loss* refers to a loss of bone in the maxilla

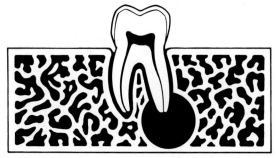

FIGURE 2–7. A unilocular corticated radiolucent lesion in the periapical location. (Modified from Eversole LR: Clinical Outline of Oral Pathology: Diagnosis and Treatment, 2d ed. Philadelphia: Lea and Febiger, 1984.)

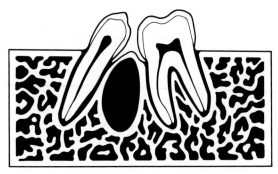

FIGURE 2–8. A unilocular corticated radiolucent lesion in the inter-radicular location. (Modified from Eversole LR: Clinical Outline of Oral Pathology: Diagnosis and Treatment, 2d ed. Philadelphia: Lea and Febiger, 1984.)

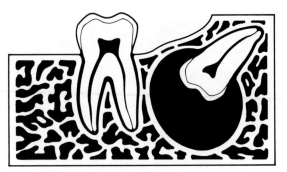

FIGURE 2–10. A unilocular corticated radiolucent lesion located in the pericoronal location. (Modified from Eversole LR: Clinical Outline of Oral Pathology: Diagnosis and Treatment, 2d ed. Philadelphia: Lea and Febiger, 1984.)

or mandible that surrounds and supports the teeth (Fig. 2–11). Alveolar bone loss appears radiolucent. Alveolar bone loss is not only seen with periodontal disease but with systemic illnesses such as diabetes, histiocytosis X and leukemia. Malignant neoplasms may also cause alveolar bone loss.

Size

Radiolucent lesions viewed on a dental radiograph can vary in size from several millimeters in diameter to several centimeters in diameter. Often the size of a lesion dictates the type of treatment necessary. Documentation of the size of a lesion is important for treatment considerations as well as for the purpose of future comparisons. Radiolucent lesions can be easily measured on a radiograph with a millimeter ruler. Figure 2–12 illustrates some common items and their respective sizes for comparison purposes.

Terms Used to Describe Radiopaque Lesions

A number of terms can be used to describe radiopaque lesions, which resist the passage of the

x-ray beam and represent osseous tissue, cartilage, enamel, dentin and cementum. Radiopaque lesions can also be described in terms of appearance, location and size.

Appearance

The appearance of a radiopaque lesion can be described as one of the following: focal opacity, target lesion, multifocal confluent, irregular, ground glass or mixed lucent-opaque. Radiopaque lesions not only occur in bone but in soft tissue as well. A radiopaque lesion located in soft tissue can be described as a soft tissue radiopacity. Examples of radiopaque lesions of the jaw are listed in Table 2–3.

Focal Opacity. The term *focal opacity* refers to a well-defined, localized radiopaque lesion on a radiograph (Fig. 2–13). Condensing osteitis is an example of a radiopaque lesion that can be described as a focal opacity.

Target Lesion. The term *target lesion* refers to a well-defined, localized radiopaque area surrounded by a uniform radiolucent halo (Fig. 2–14). A benign cementoblastoma is an example of a radiopacity that can be described as a target lesion.

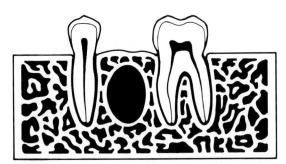

FIGURE 2–9. A unilocular corticated radiolucent lesion in the edentulous zone. (Modified from Eversole LR: Clinical Outline of Oral Pathology: Diagnosis and Treatment, 2d ed. Philadelphia: Lea and Febiger, 1984.)

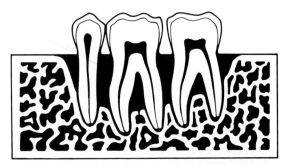

FIGURE 2–11. A radiolucent area caused by alveolar bone loss. (Modified from Eversole LR: Clinical Outline of Oral Pathology: Diagnosis and Treatment, 2d ed. Philadelphia: Lea and Febiger, 1984.)

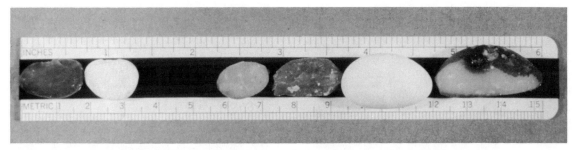

FIGURE 2–12. Beans and nuts can be used to illustrate sizes of lesions.

Multifocal Confluent. A *multifocal confluent* radiopaque pattern can be described as multiple radiopacities that appear to overlap or flow together (Fig. 2–15). Diseases such as osteitis deformans and florid osseous dysplasia exhibit a multifocal confluent radiopaque pattern. Multifocal radiopacities that involve multiple quadrants of the jaws usually represent benign fibro-osseous disorders.

Irregular, Ill-Defined. A radiopacity may exhibit an *irregular, ill-defined* pattern (Fig. 2–16). Irregular radiopacities may represent a malignant condition. Examples of irregular, ill-defined radiopaque lesions include osteosarcoma and chondrosarcoma.

Ground Glass. A *ground-glass* appearance of bone can be described as a granular or pebbled radiopacity that resembles pulverized glass (Fig. 2–17). A ground-glass radiopacity is often said to resemble the appearance or texture of an orange peel. Diseases such as fibrous dysplasia, osteitis deformans and osteopetrosis may radiographically exhibit a ground-glass or orange-peel appearance.

Mixed Lucent-Opaque. A *mixed lucent-opaque* lesion exhibits both a radiopaque and radiolucent component (Fig. 2–18). Mixed lucent-opaque lesions often represent calcifying tumors. Many such tumors appear as a radiolucent area with central opaque flecks or calcifications. With time, as the mineralization progresses, a predominantly radiolucent lesion with radiopaque flecks becomes more and more radiopaque. An example of a mixed lucent-opaque lesion is a compound odontoma.

Soft Tissue Opacity. A *soft tissue opacity* appears as a well-defined, radiopaque area located in soft tissue (Fig. 2–19). A sialolith (sali-

TABLE 2–3. Radiopaque Lesions of the Jaws

Focal Opacities	Irregular Radiopacities
Periapical cemental dysplasia*	Osteosarcoma*
Condensing osteitis	Chondrosarcoma*
Sclerotic bone	Metastatic carcinoma*
Target lesions	**Soft Tissue Radiopacities**
Benign cementoblastoma	Sialolithiasis
Complex odontoma	Calcified lymph nodes
	Foreign bodies
Multifocal Confluent Radiopacities	Myositis ossificans
Osteitis deformans	**Ground-Glass Radiopacities**
Florid osseous dysplasia	Fibrous dysplasia
Gardner's syndrome	Osteitis deformans
	Osteopetrosis
Mixed Lucent-Opaque Lesions	Hyperparathyroidism
Adenomatoid odontogenic tumor	
Calcifying epithelial odontogenic tumor	
Ameloblastic fibroma	
Ameloblastic fibro-odontoma	
Compound odontoma	
Ossifying/cementifying fibroma	
Peripical cemental dysplasia	
Calcifying and keratinizing epithelial odontogenic cyst	

* Indicates the lesion may also appear with a radiolucent component.

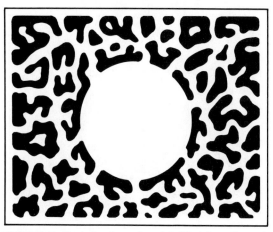

FIGURE 2–13. A focal opacity. (Modified from Eversole LR: Clinical Outline of Oral Pathology: Diagnosis and Treatment, 2d ed. Philadelphia: Lea and Febiger, 1984.)

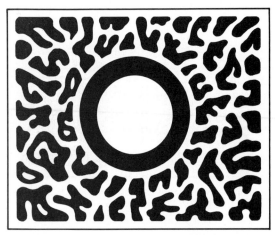

FIGURE 2–14. A target lesion. (Modified from Eversole LR: Clinical Outline of Oral Pathology: Diagnosis and Treatment, 2d ed. Philadelphia: Lea and Febiger, 1984.)

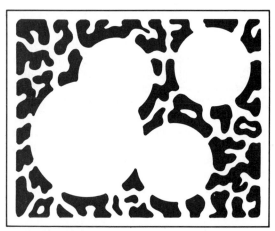

FIGURE 2–15. A multifocal confluent radiopacity. (Modified from Eversole LR: Clinical Outline of Oral Pathology: Diagnosis and Treatment, 2d ed. Philadelphia: Lea and Febiger, 1984.)

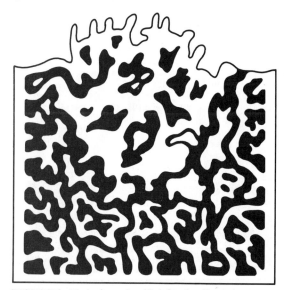

FIGURE 2–16. An irregular, ill-defined radiopaque pattern. (Modified from Eversole LR: Clinical Outline of Oral Pathology: Diagnosis and Treatment, 2d ed. Philadelphia: Lea and Febiger, 1984.)

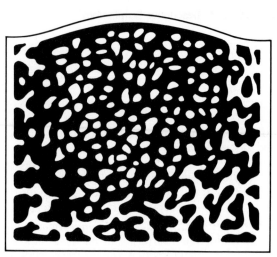

FIGURE 2–17. A ground-glass radiopacity. (Modified from Eversole LR: Clinical Outline of Oral Pathology: Diagnosis and Treatment, 2d ed. Philadelphia: Lea and Febiger, 1984.)

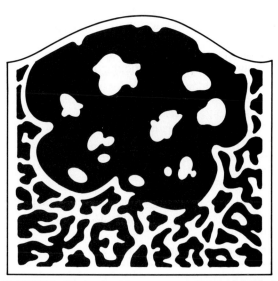

FIGURE 2–18. A mixed lucent-opaque lesion. (Modified from Eversole LR: Clinical Outline of Oral Pathology: Diagnosis and Treatment, 2d ed. Philadelphia: Lea and Febiger, 1984.)

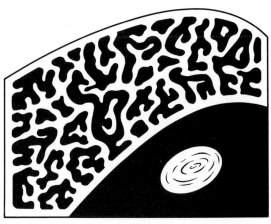

FIGURE 2–19. A soft tissue opacity. (Modified from Eversole LR: Clinical Outline of Oral Pathology: Diagnosis and Treatment, 2d ed. Philadelphia: Lea and Febiger, 1984.)

vary stone) or a calcified lymph node is an example of a soft tissue opacity.

Location

Like radiolucent lesions, radiopaque lesions can also be described in terms of location. The location of a lesion is important for communication and documentation purposes. Radiopaque lesions may appear in the same places as radiolucent lesions—in the periapical, inter-radicular, edentulous or pericoronal location. Examples of radiopaque lesions and their most common locations can be found in Table 2–4.

Periapical Location. The term *periapical* refers to a radiopaque lesion located around the apex of a tooth (Fig. 2–20). An example of a periapical radiopacity is benign cementoblastoma.

Inter-radicular Location. The term *inter-radicular* refers to a lesion located between the roots of adjacent teeth (Fig. 2–21). An example of a radiopaque lesion that would be expected to be found in the inter-radicular location is sclerotic bone.

Edentulous Zone. The term *edentulous zone* refers to a radiopaque lesion located in an area without teeth such as the complex odontoma (Fig. 2–22). A variety of radiopaque lesions may occur in the edentulous zone.

Pericoronal Location. The term *pericoronal* refers to a radiopaque lesion located around the crown of an impacted tooth (Fig. 2–23). An adenomatoid odontogenic tumor is an

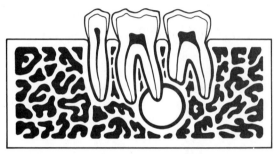

FIGURE 2–20. A radiopaque target lesion in the periapical location. (Modified from Eversole LR: Clinical Outline of Oral Pathology: Diagnosis and Treatment, 2d ed. Philadelphia: Lea and Febiger, 1984.)

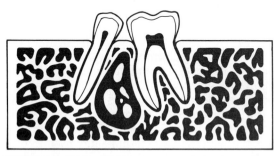

FIGURE 2–21. A mixed lucent-opaque lesion in the inter-radicular location. (Modified from Eversole LR: Clinical Outline of Oral Pathology: Diagnosis and Treatment, 2d ed. Philadelphia: Lea and Febiger, 1984.)

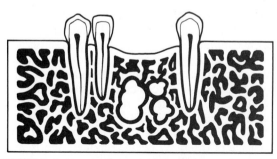

FIGURE 2–22. Multifocal confluent radiopacities in the edentulous zone. (Modified from Eversole LR: Clinical Outline of Oral Pathology: Diagnosis and Treatment, 2d ed. Philadelphia: Lea and Febiger, 1984.)

TABLE 2–4. Locations of Radiopaque Lesions

Periapical Radiopacities	Pericoronal Radiopacities
Periapical cemental dysplasia†	Adenomatoid odontogenic tumor*†
Condensing osteitis	Calcifying epithelial odontogenic tumor*†
Benign cementoblastoma	Ameloblastic fibro-odontoma
Inter-radicular Radiopacities	Compound odontoma*
	Multifocal Radiopacities
Sclerotic bone	Osteitis deformans
Calcifying and keratinizing epithelial odontogenic cyst†	Florid osseous dysplasia
Adenomatoid odontogenic tumor*†	Gardner's syndrome
	Fibrous dysplasia
Compound odontoma*	Osteopetrosis
Ossifying/cementifying fibroma†	**No Specific Location**
Edentulous Zone	Osteosarcoma†
	Chondrosarcoma†
Complex odontoma	Metastatic carcinoma†
Calcifying epithelial odontogenic tumor*†	
Ossifying/cementifying fibroma*†	

* Indicates the lesion may exhibit more than one location.
† Indicates the lesion may also appear with a radiolucent component.

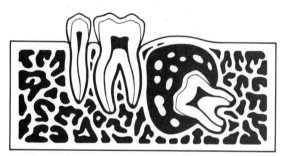

FIGURE 2–23. A mixed lucent-opaque lesion in the pericoronal location. (Modified from Eversole LR: Clinical Outline of Oral Pathology: Diagnosis and Treatment, 2d ed. Philadelphia: Lea and Febiger, 1984.)

example of a mixed lucent-opaque lesion seen in the pericoronal location.

Size

Radiopaque lesions can vary in size from several millimeters to several centimeters in diameter and can be easily measured on a radiograph with a ruler. Documentation of the size of a lesion is important for treatment decisions as well as for comparative purposes.

SUMMARY

In order to interpret dental radiographs, the dental professional must be able to accurately describe what is seen on a radiograph. The use of descriptive terminology allows the dental professional to intelligently describe and discuss what is seen on a radiograph. Descriptive terminology is important for communication and documentation purposes.

To communicate with other professionals as well as patients, the dental professional must be familiar with the basic terminology used in oral radiography. The dental professional should be familiar with the definitions and use of the general terms such as *radiograph, x-ray, radiolucent* and *radiopaque*. The term *radiograph* refers to the actual film exposed, the term *x-ray* refers to the beam of energy or radiation. The terms should not be used interchangeably. The term *radiolucent* refers to areas of a radiograph which appear dark or black. Radiolucent structures lack density and permit the passage of the x-ray beam. Air spaces and soft tissues appear radiolucent. The term *radiopaque* refers to areas of a radiograph that appear light or white. Radiopaque structures are dense and resist the passage of the x-ray beam. Enamel, dentin and bone appear radiopaque.

In addition to general terms, several terms are used to describe lesions. All lesions viewed on a radiograph should be documented and described in terms of appearance, location and size. In order to play an important role in the interpretation of dental radiographs, dental professionals must have a working knowledge of the key words in this chapter so they can describe the appearance, location and size of radiolucent and radiopaque lesions.

Bibliography

Eversole LR: Radiolucent lesions of the jaws. *In* Clinical Outline of Oral Pathology: Diagnosis and Treatment, 3d ed., pp 226–89. Philadelphia: Lea and Febiger, 1992.

Eversole LR: Radiopaque lesions of the jaws. *In* Clinical Outline of Oral Pathology: Diagnosis and Treatment, 3d ed., pp. 290–326. Philadelphia: Lea and Febiger, 1992.

Gibilisco JA: Odontogenic tumors. *In* Stafne's Oral Radiographic Diagnosis, pp 180–209. Philadelphia: WB Saunders, 1985.

Gibilisco JA: Cysts of the jaws. *In* Stafne's Oral Radiographic Diagnosis, pp 159–179. Philadelphia: WB Saunders, 1985.

Goaz PW and White SC: Cysts of the jaws. *In* Oral Radiology Principles and Interpretation, 2d ed., pp. 486–500. St Louis: CV Mosby, 1987.

Goaz PW, White SC. Benign tumors of the jaws. *In* Oral Radiology Principles and Interpretation, 2d ed., pp 520–43. St Louis: CV Mosby, 1987.

Hubar JS. Survey of dental radiographic terms. Oral Surg Oral Path Oral Med 69:530–31, 1990.

Langland OE, Sippy FH, and Langlais RP: Principles of interpretation of pathologic conditions. *In* Textbook of Dental Radiography, 2d ed., pp 367–79. Springfield, IL: Charles C Thomas, 1984.

Regezi JA and Sciubba JJ: Clinical overview—jaw lesions. *In* Oral Pathology Clinical-Pathologic Correlations, pp O/69–071. Philadelphia: WB Saunders, 1989.

Regezi JA and Sciubba JJ: Clinical overview—odontogenic tumors. *In* Oral Pathology Clinical-Pathologic Correlations, pp 079–085. Philadelphia: WB Saunders, 1989.

Regezi JA and Sciubba JJ: Clinical overview—nonodontogenic tumors. *In* Oral Pathology Clinical-Pathologic Correlations, pp 085–091. Philadelphia: WB Saunders, 1989.

Shafer WG, et al.:Cysts and tumors of odontogenic origin. *In* A Textbook of Oral Pathology, 4th ed., pp 258–311. Philadelphia: WB Saunders, 1983.

Wood NK and Goaz PW: Periapical radiolucencies *In* Differential Diagnosis of Oral Lesions, 4th ed., pp 303–39. St. Louis: CV Mosby, 1991.

Wood NK and Goaz PW: Pericoronal radiolucencies. *In* Differential Diagnosis of Oral Lesions, 4th ed., pp 340–60. St. Louis: CV Mosby, 1991.

Wood NK and Goaz PW: Multilocular radiolucencies. *In* Differential Diagnosis of Oral Lesions, 4th ed., pp 406–28. St. Louis: CV Mosby, 1991.

Wood NK and Goaz PW: Periapical radiopacities. *In* Differential Diagnosis of Oral Lesions, 4th ed., pp 548–69. St. Louis: CV Mosby, 1991.

Wood NK and Goaz PW: Generalized radiopacities. *In* Differential Diagnosis of Oral Lesions, 4th ed., pp 604–13. St. Louis: CV Mosby, 1991.

QUIZ QUESTIONS

"What Can This Be?"

1. Describe the lesion illustrated in Figure 2–24 in terms of the following:

   • Appearance:_____
   • Location:_____
   • Size:_____

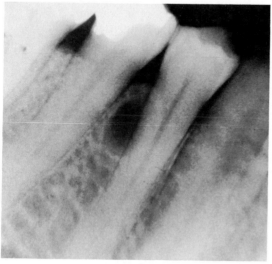

FIGURE 2–24.

2. Describe the lesion illustrated in Figure 2–25 in terms of the following:

   • Appearance:_____
   • Location:_____
   • Size:_____

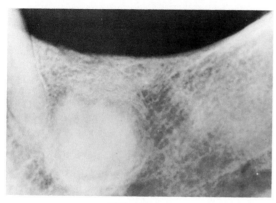

FIGURE 2–25.

3. Describe the lesion illustrated in Figure 2–26 in terms of the following:

   • Appearance:_____
   • Location:_____
   • Size:_____

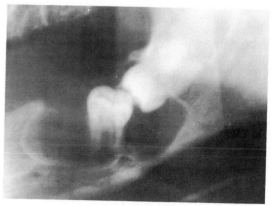

FIGURE 2–26.

Matching

Match the following terms with the proper definitions.

___ **4.** ground glass

___ **5.** inter-radicular

___ **6.** radiopaque

___ **7.** pericoronal

___ **8.** corticated

a. the location of a lesion surrounding the crown of an impacted tooth

b. the location of a lesion found between the roots of adjacent teeth

c. the location of a lesion found surrounding the apex of a tooth

d. a descriptive term for a radiopaque lesion that resembles an orange peel or has a granular appearance

e. a term for structures that are dense and absorb or resist the passage of the x-ray beam

Continued on following page

Continued

___ **9.** target lesion

___ **10.** periapical

f. a term for the periphery of a lesion surrounded by dense cortical bone

g. a descriptive term for a radiopaque lesion that exhibits a well-demarcated, localized area

with a surrounding radiolucent ring

h. a term for structures that lack density and permit the passage of the x-ray beam with little or no resistance

CHAPTER THREE

Normal Anatomy (Periapical Films)

Objectives

After completion of this chapter, the student will be able to:

▶ State the difference between cortical and cancellous bone.

▶ Define the general terms that describe prominences, spaces and depressions in bone.

▶ Identify and describe the normal anatomic landmarks of the maxilla on a human skull.

▶ Identify and describe the normal anatomic landmarks of the maxilla viewed on dental radiographs.

▶ Identify and describe the normal anatomic landmarks of the mandible on a human skull.

▶ Identify and describe the normal anatomic landmarks of the mandible viewed on dental radiographs.

▶ Identify and describe the radiographic appearance of tooth anatomy.

▶ Identify each normal radiographic landmark of the maxilla and mandible as either radiolucent or radiopaque.

▶ Identify each normal anatomic landmark of a tooth as radiolucent or radiopaque.

Key Words

Alveolar bone	Incisive foramen	Nasal septum
Alveolar crest	Inferior nasal conchae	Nutrient canals
Anterior nasal spine	Internal oblique ridge	Periodontal ligament space
Canal	Inverted "Y"	Process
Cancellous	Lamina dura	Pulp cavity
Coronoid process	Lateral fossa	Ridge
Cortical	Lingual foramen	Septum
Dentin	Mandibular canal	Sinus
Dentino-enamel junction	Maxillary sinus	Spine
Enamel	Maxillary tuberosity	Submandibular fossa
External oblique ridge	Median palatal suture	Superior foramina of the incisive canal
Floor of nasal cavity	Mental foramen	Suture
Foramen	Mental fossa	Tubercle
Fossa	Mental ridge	Tuberosity
Genial tubercles	Mylohyoid ridge	Zygoma
Hamulus	Nasal cavity	Zygomatic process of the maxilla

Dental professionals must be able to recognize normal anatomic landmarks viewed on periapical films. The recognition of normal radiographic landmarks enables the dental professional to accurately mount dental films and interpret dental radiographs. Without a working knowledge of anatomy, the dental professional may mistake normal anatomic structures for pathologic conditions.

In order to interpret dental radiographs and identify anatomic landmarks, the dental professional must have a thorough knowledge of the anatomy of the maxilla and mandible. Each normal anatomic landmark seen on a periapical radiograph corresponds to what is seen on the human skull. If dental professionals know the anatomy of the maxilla and mandible and surrounding structures, they can identify the normal anatomy seen on a radiograph. In addition to memorizing the names and locations of the bony landmarks of the maxilla and mandible, dental professionals must train their eyes to recognize the subtle radiographic images that represent these normal anatomic structures.

The normal anatomy presented in Chapter 3 is designed to enable the dental professional to view each anatomic structure of the maxilla and mandible as it appears in a photograph of the human skull, a diagrammatic sketch and a periapical radiograph.

DEFINITIONS OF GENERAL TERMS

A number of general terms exist that can be used to describe the anatomy of the bones of the skull. Terms describing the types of bone, bony prominences and bony spaces and depressions can be used to characterize areas of the maxilla and mandible normally viewed on periapical radiographs. General terms can be utilized by the dental professional to describe areas of normal anatomy viewed on dental radiographs.

Types of Bone

The composition of bone in the human body can be described as either cortical or cancellous.

Cortical Bone

The term *cortical* is derived from the Latin word *cortex* and means "outer layer." Cortical bone, also referred to as compact bone, is the dense outer layer of bone (Fig. 3–1). Cortical bone

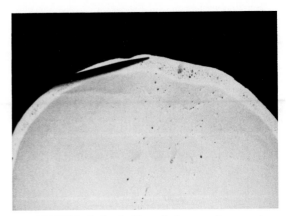

FIGURE 3–1. Cortical bone is dense and compact.

resists the passage of the x-ray beam and appears *radiopaque* on a radiograph. The inferior border of the mandible is composed of cortical bone and appears radiopaque (Fig. 3–2).

Cancellous Bone

The term *cancellous* is also derived from Latin and means "arranged like a lattice." Cancellous bone is the soft spongy bone that is located between two layers of dense cortical bone (Fig. 3–3). Cancellous bone is composed of numerous bony trabeculae that form a lattice-like network

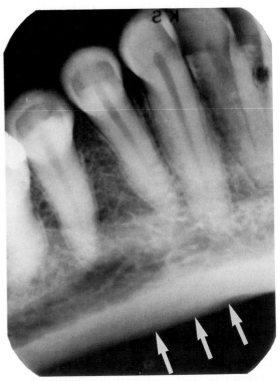

FIGURE 3–2. Cortical bone appears very radiopaque on a dental radiograph.

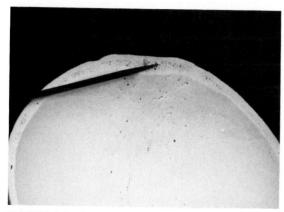

FIGURE 3–3. Cancellous or spongy bone is composed of numerous trabecular spaces.

of intercommunicating spaces filled with bone marrow. The trabeculae, actual pieces of bone, resist the passage of the x-ray beam and appear radiopaque; in contrast, the marrow spaces permit the passage of the x-ray beam and appear radiolucent. The larger the trabeculations, the more radiolucent the area of cancellous bone appears. Cancellous bone appears predominantly *radiolucent* (Fig. 3–4).

Prominences of Bone

Prominences of bone are comprised of dense, *cortical* bone and appear *radiopaque* on dental radiographs. There are five terms that can be used to describe the prominences of bone viewed in maxillary and mandibular periapical radiographs: process, ridge, spine, tubercle and tuberosity.

PROCESS   A marked prominence or projection of bone.

Example: coronoid process (Fig. 3–5).

RIDGE   A linear prominence or projection of bone.

Example: internal oblique ridge (Fig. 3–6).

SPINE   A sharp, thorn-like projection of bone.

Example: anterior nasal spine (Fig. 3–7).

TUBERCLE   A small bump or nodule of bone.

Example: genial tubercles (Fig. 3–8).

TUBEROSITY   A rounded prominence of bone.

Example: maxillary tuberosity (Fig. 3–9).

Spaces and Depressions in Bone

Spaces and depressions in bone do not resist the passage of the x-ray beam and appear *radiolucent* on dental radiographs. There are four terms that can be used to describe the spaces and depressions in bone viewed in maxillary and mandibular periapical radiographs: canal, foramen, fossa and sinus.

CANAL   A tube-like passageway through bone that houses nerves and blood vessels.

Example: mandibular canal (Fig. 3–10).

FORAMEN   An opening or hole in bone that permits the passage of nerves and blood vessels.

Example: mental foramen (Fig. 3–11).

FOSSA   A broad and shallow scooped-out or depressed area of bone.

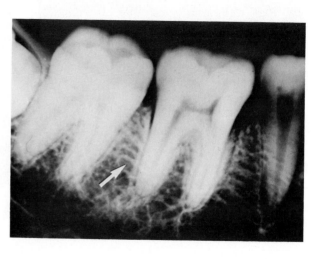

FIGURE 3–4. Cancellous bone appears predominantly radiolucent.

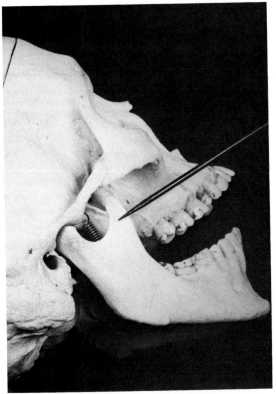

FIGURE 3–5. A process is a marked projection of bone.

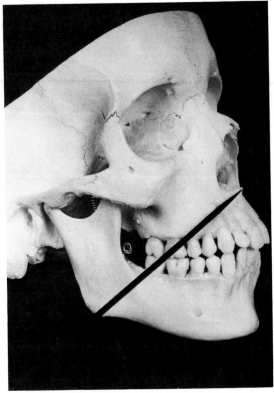

FIGURE 3–7. A spine is a sharp projection of bone.

Example: submandibular fossa (Fig. 3–12).

SINUS   A hollow space, cavity or recess in bone.

Example: maxillary sinus (Fig. 3–13).

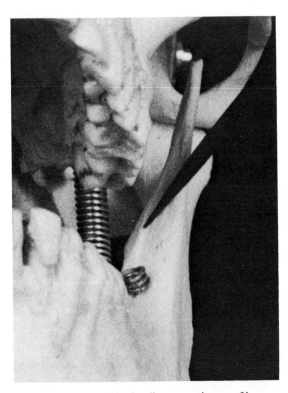

FIGURE 3–6. A ridge is a linear prominence of bone.

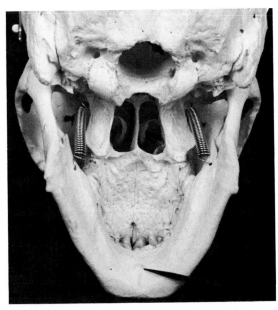

FIGURE 3–8. A tubercle is a tiny bump of bone.

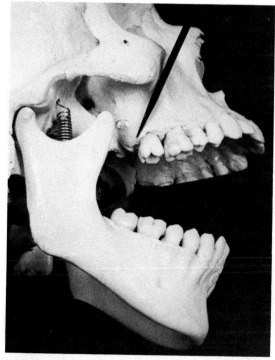

FIGURE 3–9. A tuberosity is a rounded prominence of bone.

Miscellaneous General Terms

Two other general terms that can be used to describe normal radiographic landmarks are septum and suture.

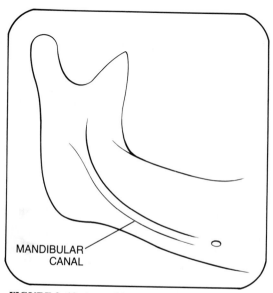

FIGURE 3–10. A canal is a passageway through bone.

MANDIBULAR CANAL

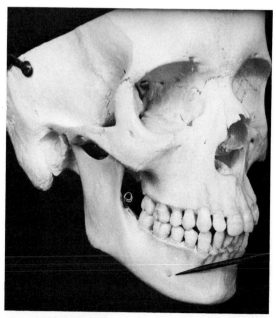

FIGURE 3–11. A foramen is a hole in bone.

SEPTUM   The term *septum* refers to a bony wall or partition that divides two spaces or cavities. A septum may be present within the space of a fossa or sinus. A bony septum appears *radiopaque,* in contrast to a space or cavity, which appears radiolucent.

Example: nasal septum (Fig. 3–14).

SUTURE   A *suture* is an immovable joint that represents a line of union between adjoining

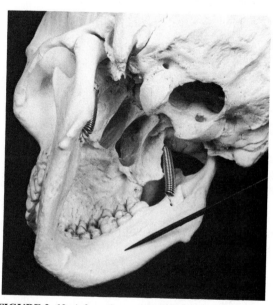

FIGURE 3–12. A fossa is a scooped-out or depressed area of bone.

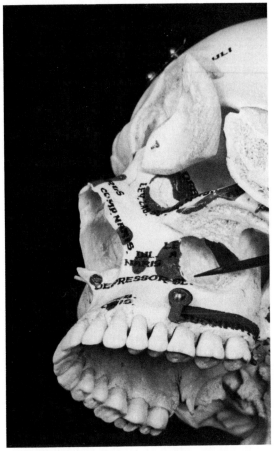

FIGURE 3–13. A sinus is a hollow cavity in bone.

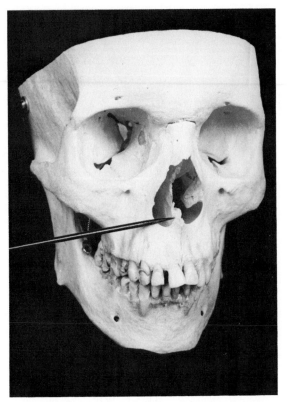

FIGURE 3–14. A septum is a bony partition.

bones of the skull. (Sutures are only found in the skull.) Radiographically, a suture appears as a thin *radiolucent* line.

Example: median palatal suture (Fig. 3–15).

NORMAL ANATOMIC LANDMARKS

Bony Landmarks of the Maxilla

The upper jaw is comprised of two paired maxillae bones (Fig. 3–16). The paired maxillae meet at the midline of the face and are often referred to as a single bone, "the maxilla." The maxilla has been described as the architectural cornerstone of the face. All of the bones of the face articulate with the maxilla, with the exception of the mandible. The maxilla forms the floor of the orbit of the eyes, the sides and floor of the nasal cavities and the hard palate. The lower border of the maxilla supports the upper teeth.

This portion of Chapter 3 reviews the bony landmarks that frequently appear in maxillary periapical radiographs.

Incisive Foramen

Description. The **incisive foramen** (also known as the nasopalatine foramen) is an opening or hole in bone located at the midline of the

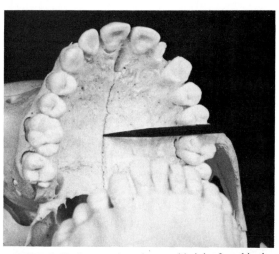

FIGURE 3–15. A suture is an immovable joint found in the skull.

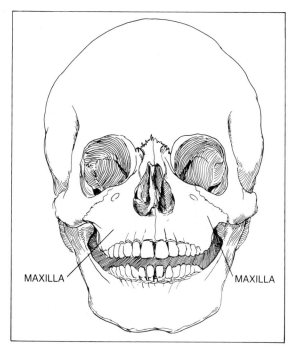

FIGURE 3–16. The paired bones of the maxilla.

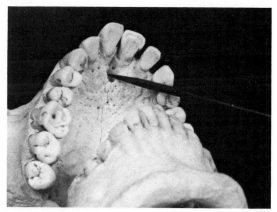

FIGURE 3–17. The incisive foramen is seen posterior to the maxillary central incisors.

anterior portion of the hard palate directly posterior to the maxillary central incisors (Fig. 3–17). The nasopalatine nerve exits the maxilla through the incisive foramen.

Radiographic Appearance. On a maxillary periapical radiograph, the incisive foramen appears as a small ovoid or round *radiolucency* located between the roots of the maxillary central incisors (Figs. 3–18 and 3–19).

Superior Foramina of the Incisive Canal

Description. The **superior foramina** (the plural of *foramen*) of the incisive canal are two tiny openings or holes in bone located on the floor of the nasal cavity (Fig. 3–20). The superior foramina represent the openings of two small canals that extend from the floor of the nasal cavity downward and medially. These two small canals join together to form the incisive canal and share a common exit, the incisive foramen. The nasopalatine nerve enters the maxilla via the superior foramina, travels through the incisive canal, and exits at the incisive foramen.

Radiographic Appearance. On a maxillary periapical radiograph, the superior foramina appear as two small, round *radiolucencies* located superior to the apices of the maxillary central incisors (Figs. 3–21 and 3–22).

Median Palatal Suture

Description. The **median palatal suture** represents the immovable joint between the two palatine processes of the maxilla. (The palatine processes of the maxilla form the major portion of the hard palate.) The median palatal suture extends from the alveolar bone between the maxillary central incisors to the posterior hard palate (Fig. 3–23).

Radiographic Appearance. On a maxillary periapical radiograph, the median palatal

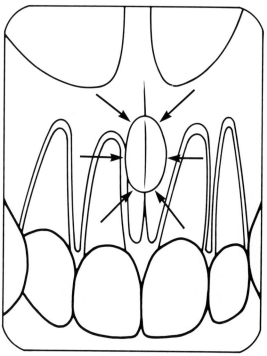

FIGURE 3–18. The incisive foramen.

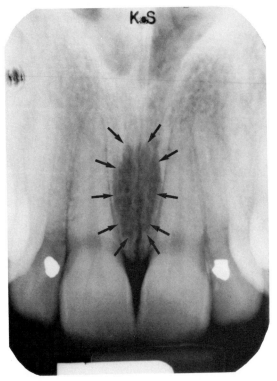

FIGURE 3–19. The incisive foramen appears radiolucent.

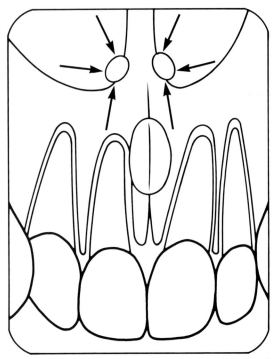

FIGURE 3–21. The superior foramina of the incisive canal.

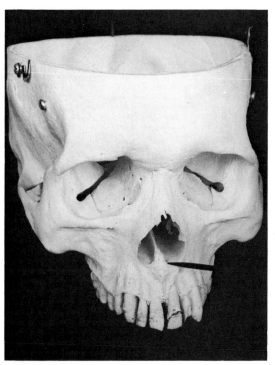

FIGURE 3–20. The superior foramina of the incisive canal are found on the floor of the nasal cavity.

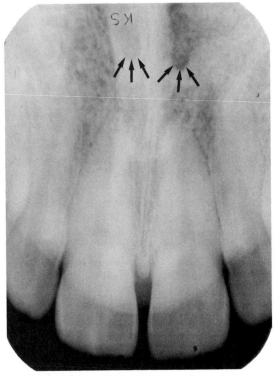

FIGURE 3–22. The superior foramina of the incisive canal appear as two small round radiolucencies.

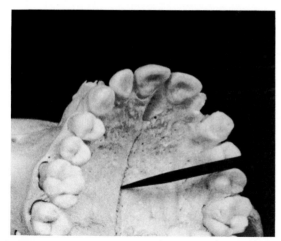

FIGURE 3–23. The median palatal suture is found between the two palatine processes of the maxilla.

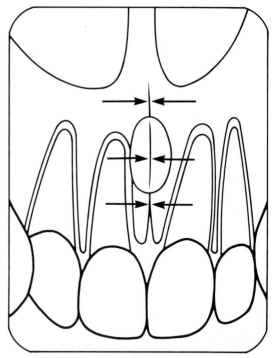

FIGURE 3–24. The median palatal suture.

suture appears as a thin *radiolucent* line between the maxillary central incisors (Figs. 3–24 and 3–25). The median palatal suture is bounded on both sides by dense cortical bone, which appears radiopaque. As the median palatal suture fuses with age, it may appear less distinct radiographically.

Lateral Fossa

Description. The **lateral fossa** (also known as the canine fossa) is a smooth depressed area of the maxilla located just inferior and medial to the infraorbital foramen between the canine and lateral incisor (Fig. 3–26).

Radiographic Appearance. On a maxillary periapical radiograph, the lateral fossa appears as a *radiolucency* between the maxillary canine and lateral incisor (Figs. 3–27 and 3–28). In some periapical radiographs, the lateral fossa may appear as a distinct radiolucency; in others, it may appear to be absent. The radiographic appearance of the lateral fossa varies depending upon the anatomy of the individual.

Nasal Cavity

Description. The **nasal cavity** (also known as the nasal fossa) is a pear-shaped compartment of bone located superior to the maxilla (Fig. 3–29). The inferior portion, or floor, of the nasal cavity is formed by the palatal processes of the maxilla and the horizontal portions of the palatine bones. The lateral walls of the nasal cavity are formed by the ethmoid and maxillae bones. The nasal cavity is divided by a bony partition, or wall, called the nasal septum.

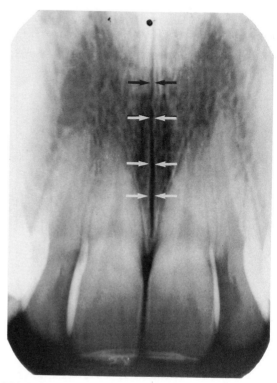

FIGURE 3–25. The median palatal suture appears as a thin radiolucent line.

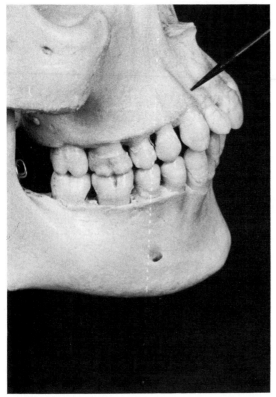

FIGURE 3–26. The lateral fossa is a depressed area of the maxilla found between the lateral incisor and the canine.

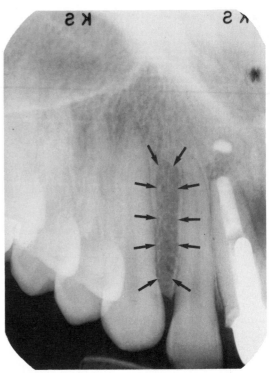

FIGURE 3–28. The lateral fossa appears as a radiolucent area between the lateral incisor and the canine.

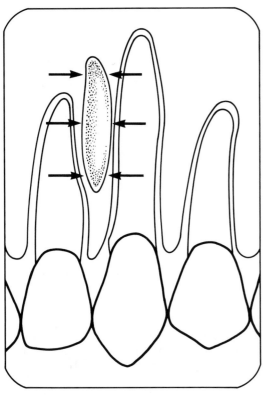

FIGURE 3–27. The lateral fossa.

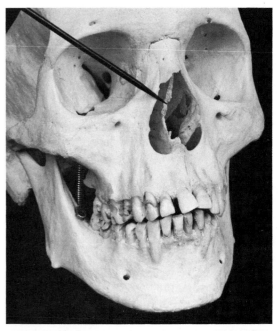

FIGURE 3–29. The nasal cavity is a pear-shaped opening of the skull found above the maxilla.

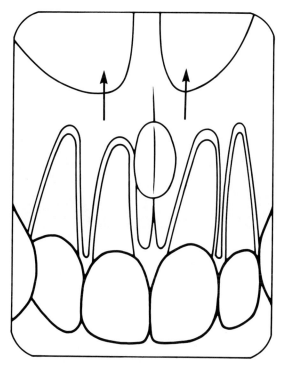

FIGURE 3–30. The nasal cavity.

Radiographic Appearance. On a maxillary periapical radiograph, the nasal cavity appears as a large *radiolucent* area above the maxillary incisors (Figs. 3–30 and 3–31).

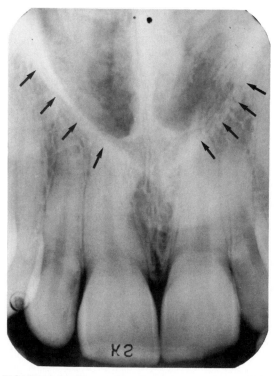

FIGURE 3–31. The nasal cavity appears as a large radiolucent area above the maxilla.

Nasal Septum

Description. The **nasal septum** is a vertical bony wall or partition that divides the nasal cavity into the right and left nasal *fossae* (the plural of *fossa*) (Fig. 3–32). The nasal septum is formed by two bones (the vomer and a portion of the ethmoid bone) and cartilage.

Radiographic Appearance. On a maxillary periapical radiograph, the nasal septum appears as a vertical *radiopaque* partition that divides the nasal cavity (Figs. 3–33 and 3–34). The nasal septum may appear superimposed over the median palatal suture.

Floor of the Nasal Cavity

Description. The **floor of the nasal cavity** is a bony wall formed by the palatal processes of the maxillae and the horizontal portions of the palatine bones (Fig. 3–35). The floor is comprised of dense cortical bone and defines the inferior border of the nasal cavity.

Radiographic Appearance. On a maxillary periapical radiograph, the floor of the nasal cavity appears as a dense *radiopaque* band of bone above the maxillary incisors (Figs. 3–36 and 3–37).

Anterior Nasal Spine

Description. The **anterior nasal spine** is a sharp projection of the maxilla located at the

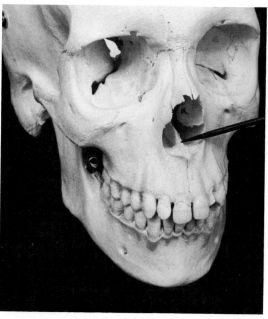

FIGURE 3–32. The nasal septum is a bony wall that divides the nasal cavity into two nasal fossae.

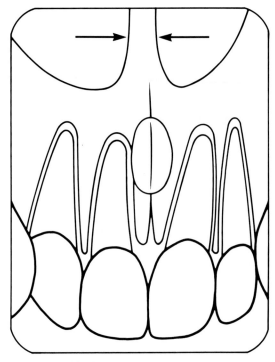

FIGURE 3–33. The nasal septum.

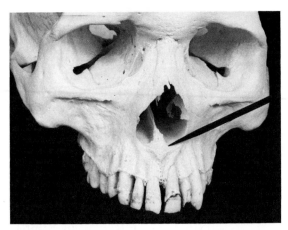

FIGURE 3–35. The floor of the nasal cavity is composed of dense cortical bone.

anterior and inferior portion of the nasal cavity (Fig. 3–38).

Radiographic Appearance. On a maxillary periapical radiograph, the anterior nasal spine appears as a V-shaped *radiopaque* area located at the intersection of the floor of the nasal cavity and the nasal septum (Figs. 3–39 and 3–40).

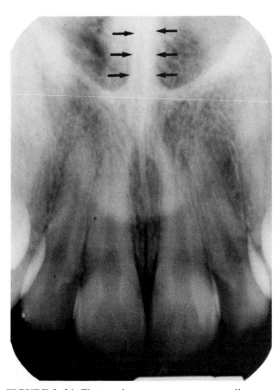

FIGURE 3–34. The nasal septum appears as a radiopaque partition that divides the nasal cavity.

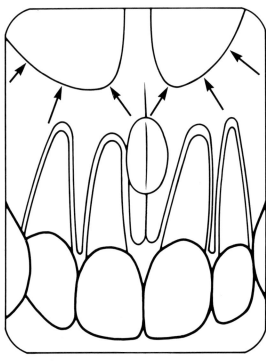

FIGURE 3–36. The floor of the nasal cavity.

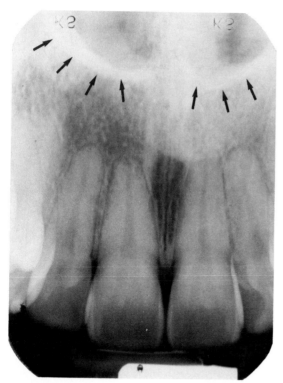

FIGURE 3–37. The floor of the nasal cavity appears as a radiopaque band.

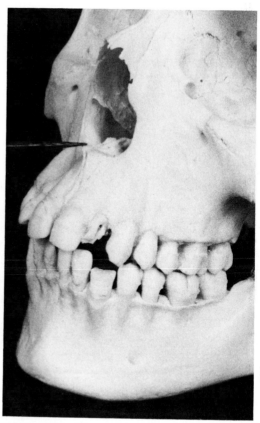

FIGURE 3–38. The anterior nasal spine is a sharp projection of bone located at the anterior inferior point of the nasal cavity.

Inferior Nasal Conchae

Description. The **inferior nasal conchae** are wafer-thin curved plates of bone that extend from the lateral walls of the nasal cavity (Fig. 3–41). The inferior nasal conchae are seen in the lower lateral portions of the nasal cavity. The term *concha* is derived from Latin and means "shell-shaped" or "scroll-shaped."

Radiographic Appearance. On a maxillary periapical radiograph, the inferior nasal conchae appear as a diffuse *radiopaque* mass or projection within the nasal cavity (Figs. 3–42 and 3–43).

Maxillary Sinus

Description. The **maxillary sinuses** are paired cavities or compartments of bone located within the maxilla (Fig. 3–44). The maxillary sinuses are located above the maxillary premolar and molar teeth. Rarely does the maxillary sinus extend anteriorly beyond the canine. At birth, the maxillary sinus is the size of a small pea. As growth takes place, the maxillary sinus expands and occupies a large portion of the maxilla. The maxillary sinus may extend to include interdental bone, molar furcation areas or the maxillary tuberosity region.

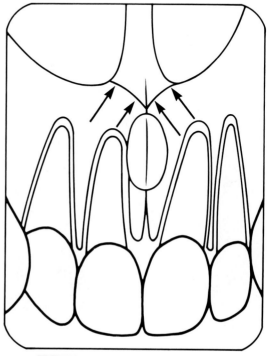

FIGURE 3–39. The anterior nasal spine.

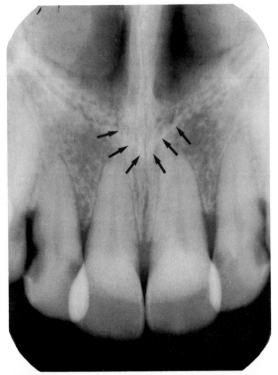

FIGURE 3–40. The anterior nasal spine appears as a V-shaped radiopacity at the midline of the floor of the nasal cavity.

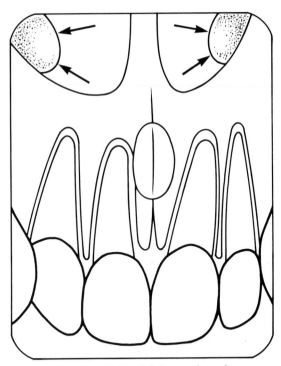

FIGURE 3–42. The inferior nasal conchae.

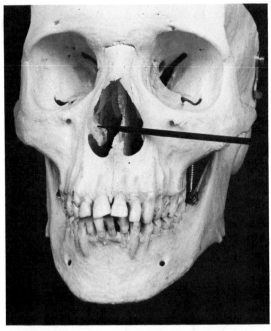

FIGURE 3–41. The inferior nasal conchae are scroll-shaped plates of bone that extend from the lateral wall of the nasal fossa.

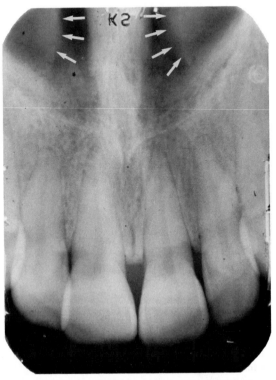

FIGURE 3–43. The inferior nasal conchae appear as diffuse radiopacities within the nasal cavity.

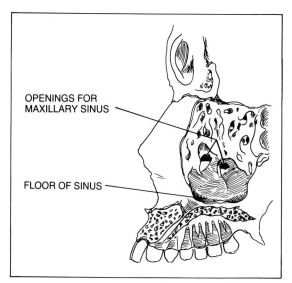

FIGURE 3–44. The maxillary sinuses are paired compartments of bone located above the maxillary posterior teeth.

Radiographic Appearance. On a maxillary periapical radiograph, the maxillary sinus appears as a *radiolucent* area located above the apices of the maxillary premolars and molars (Figs. 3–45 and 3–46). The floor of the maxillary sinus is composed of dense cortical bone and appears as a radiopaque line.

Maxillary Sinus-Septa

Description. Bony septa may be seen within the maxillary sinus. **Septa** (the plural of *septum*) are bony walls or partitions that appear to divide the maxillary sinus into compartments (Fig. 3–47).

Radiographic Appearance. On a maxillary periapical radiograph, the septa appear as *radiopaque* lines within the maxillary sinus (Figs. 3–48 and 3–49). In some periapical radiographs, the septa appear as distinct radiopaque lines; in others, no septa are present. The presence and number of bony septa within a maxillary sinus vary based on the anatomy of the individual.

Maxillary Sinuses and Nutrient Canals

Description. Nutrient canals may be seen within the maxillary sinuses. **Nutrient canals** are tiny tube-like passageways through bone that house blood vessels and nerves supplying the maxillary teeth and interdental areas (Fig. 3–50).

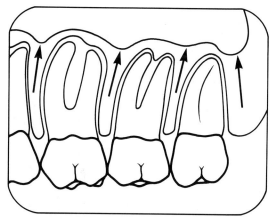

FIGURE 3–45. The maxillary sinus.

Radiographic Appearance. On a maxillary periapical radiograph, a nutrient canal appears as a narrow *radiolucent* band bounded by two thin radiopaque lines (Figs. 3–51 and 3–52). The radiopaque lines represent cortical bone, which comprises the walls of the canal.

Inverted "Y"

Description. The **Inverted "Y"** refers to the intersection of the maxillary sinus and the nasal cavity as viewed on a dental radiograph.

Radiographic Appearance. On a maxillary periapical radiograph, the inverted "Y" appears as a *radiopaque* upside-down "Y" formed by the intersection of the lateral wall of the nasal fossa and the anterior border of the maxillary sinus (Figs. 3–53 and 3–54). Both the lateral wall of the nasal cavity and the anterior border of the maxillary sinus are comprised of dense cortical bone and appear as a radiopaque line or band. The inverted "Y" is located above the maxillary canine.

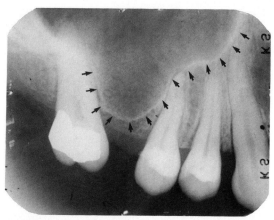

FIGURE 3–46. The maxillary sinus appears as a radiolucent area above the maxillary posterior teeth.

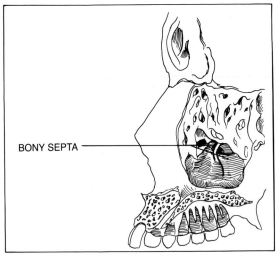

FIGURE 3–47. Septa are bony walls within the maxillary sinus.

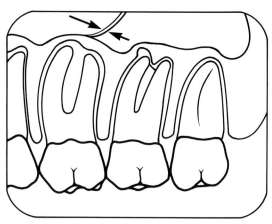

FIGURE 3–50. Nutrient canals in the maxillary sinus are tiny passageways through bone.

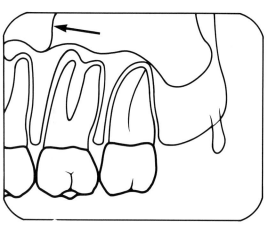

FIGURE 3–48. Septa within the maxillary sinus.

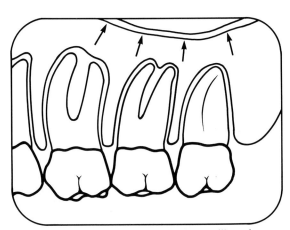

FIGURE 3–51. Nutrient canals in the maxillary sinus.

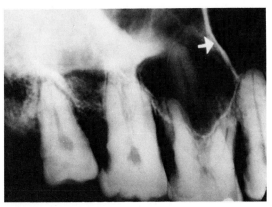

FIGURE 3–49. Septa within the maxillary sinus appear as radiopaque lines.

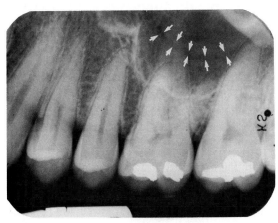

FIGURE 3–52. Nutrient canals appear as narrow, radiolucent lines.

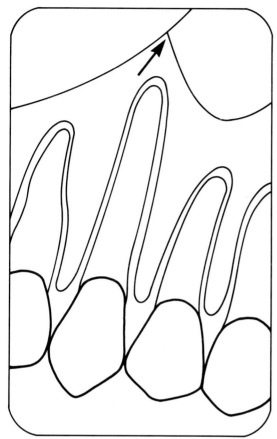

FIGURE 3–53. The inverted "*Y*" refers to the intersection of the anterior wall of the maxillary sinus and the lateral wall of the nasal cavity.

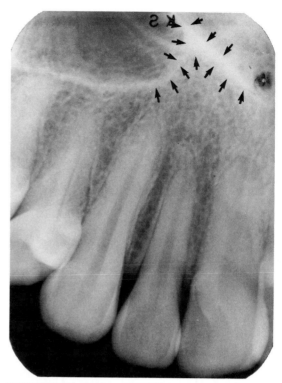

FIGURE 3–54. The inverted "*Y*" appears as a radiopaque, upside-down "*Y.*"

Maxillary Tuberosity

Description. The **maxillary tuberosity** is a rounded prominence of bone that extends posterior to the third molar region (Fig. 3–55). Blood vessels and nerves enter the maxilla in this region and supply the posterior teeth.

Radiographic Appearance. On a maxillary periapical radiograph, the maxillary tuberosity appears as a *radiopaque* bulge distal to the third molar region (Figs. 3–56 and 3–57).

Hamulus

Description. The **hamulus** (also known as the hamular process) is a small hook-like projection of bone that extends from the medial pterygoid plate of the sphenoid bone (Fig. 3–58). The hamulus is located posterior to the maxillary tuberosity region.

Radiographic Appearance. On a maxillary periapical radiograph, the hamulus appears as a *radiopaque* hook-like projection posterior to the maxillary tuberosity area (Figs. 3–59 and

3–60). The radiographic appearance of the hamulus varies in length, shape and density.

Zygomatic Process of the Maxilla

Description. The **zygomatic process of the maxilla** is a bony projection of the maxilla that articulates with the zygoma or malar (cheek) bone (Fig. 3–61). The zygomatic process of the maxilla is comprised of dense cortical bone.

Radiographic Appearance. On a maxillary periapical radiograph, the zygomatic process of the maxilla appears as a J- or U-shaped *radiopacity* located superior to the maxillary first molar region (Figs. 3–62 and 3–63).

Zygoma

Description. The **zygoma** or cheek bone (also referred to as the malar or zygomatic bone) articulates with the zygomatic process of the maxilla (Fig. 3–64). The zygoma is comprised of dense cortical bone.

Radiographic Appearance. On a maxillary periapical radiograph, the zygoma appears as a diffuse *radiopaque* band that extends pos-

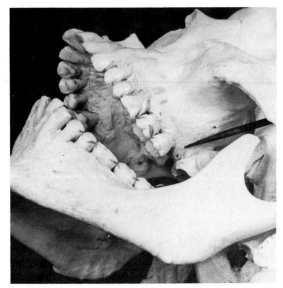

FIGURE 3–55. The maxillary tuberosity is a rounded prominence of bone posterior to the third molar region.

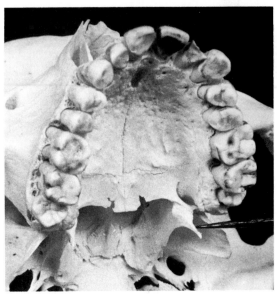

FIGURE 3–58. The hamulus is a hook-like projection of bone that extends from the medial pterygoid plate.

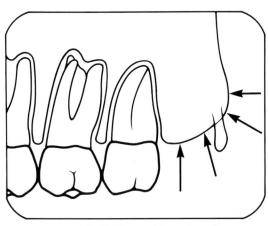

FIGURE 3–56. The maxillary tuberosity.

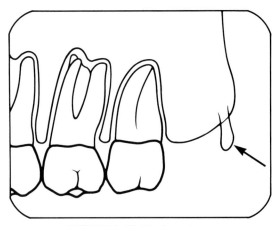

FIGURE 3–59. The hamulus.

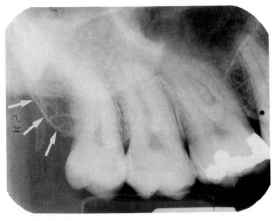

FIGURE 3–57. The maxillary tuberosity appears as a radiopaque bulge distal to the third molar region.

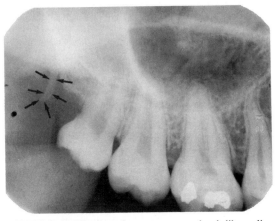

FIGURE 3–60. The hamulus appears as a hook-like radiopacity distal to the maxillary tuberosity area.

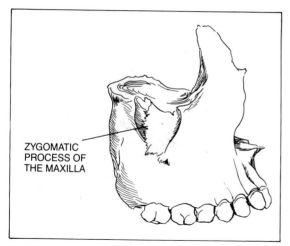

FIGURE 3–61. The zygomatic process of the maxilla is a small portion of the maxilla that articulates with the zygoma.

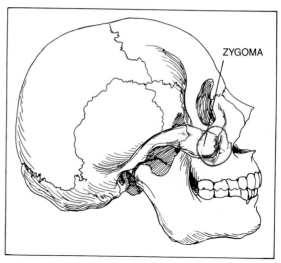

FIGURE 3–64. The zygoma (or the cheekbone) articulates with the zygomatic process of the maxilla.

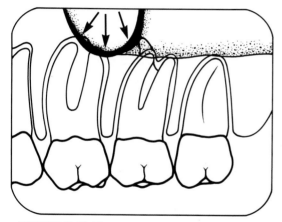

FIGURE 3–62. The zygomatic process of the maxilla.

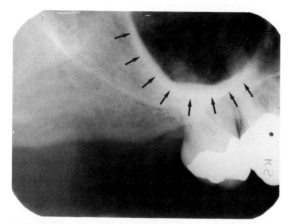

FIGURE 3–63. The zygomatic process of the maxilla appears as a J- or U-shaped radiopacity superior to the maxillary molars.

teriorly from the zygomatic process of the maxilla (Figs. 3–65 and 3–66).

Bony Landmarks of the Mandible

The mandible, or lower jaw, is the largest and strongest bone of the face. The mandible can be divided into three main parts: the ramus, the body and the alveolar process (Fig. 3–67).

RAMUS The ramus is the vertical portion of the mandible found posterior to the third molar. The mandible has two rami (the plural of *ramus*), one on each side (Fig. 3–68).

BODY The body of the mandible is the horizontal U-shaped portion that extends from ramus to ramus (Fig. 3–69).

ALVEOLAR PROCESS The alveolar process of the mandible is the bone that encases and supports the teeth (Fig. 3–70).

This portion of Chapter 3 reviews the bony landmarks that frequently appear in mandibular periapical radiographs.

Genial Tubercles

Description. The **genial tubercles** are tiny bumps of bone that serve as attachment sites for the genioglossus and geniohyoid muscles (Fig. 3–71). The genial tubercles are located on the lingual aspect of the mandible.

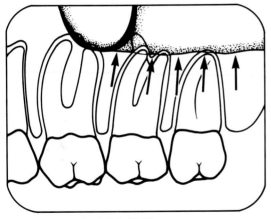

FIGURE 3–65. The zygoma.

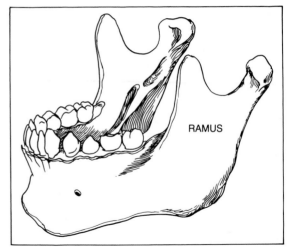

FIGURE 3–68. The ramus of the mandible.

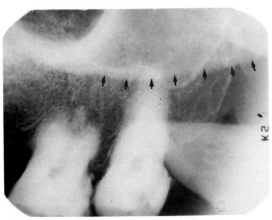

FIGURE 3–66. The zygoma appears as a diffuse radiopaque band that extends distally from the zygomatic process of the maxilla.

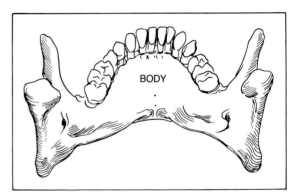

FIGURE 3–69. The body of the mandible.

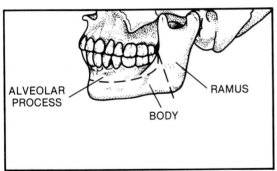

FIGURE 3–67. The mandible.

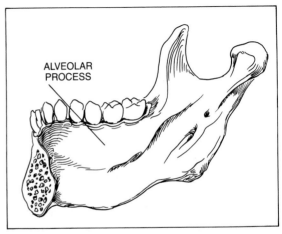

FIGURE 3–70. The alveolar process of the mandible.

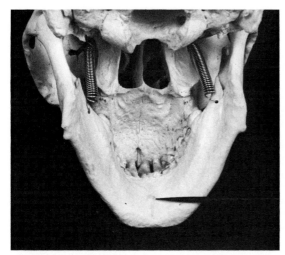

FIGURE 3–71. The genial tubercles are tiny bumps of bone seen at the midline on the lingual surface of the mandible.

Radiographic Appearance. On a mandibular periapical radiograph, the genial tubercles appear as a ring-shaped *radiopacity* below the apices of the mandibular incisors (Figs. 3–72 and 3–73).

Lingual Foramen

Description. The **lingual foramen** is a tiny opening or hole in bone located on the internal surface of the mandible (Fig. 3–74). The lingual foramen is located near the midline and is surrounded by the genial tubercles.

Radiographic Appearance. On a mandibular periapical radiograph, the lingual foramen appears as a small *radiolucent* dot located inferior to the apices of the mandibular incisors (Figs. 3–75 and 3–76). The lingual foramen is surrounded by the genial tubercles, which appear as a radiopaque ring.

Nutrient Canals

Description. Nutrient canals are tube-like passageways through bone that house nerves and blood vessels supplying the teeth. Interdental nutrient canals are most often seen in the anterior mandible, a region that typically exhibits thin bone.

Radiographic Appearance. On a mandibular periapical radiograph, nutrient canals appear as vertical *radiolucent* lines (Figs. 3–77 and 3–78). Radiographically, nutrient canals are readily seen in areas of thin bone. In the edentulous mandible, nutrient canals may appear more prominent.

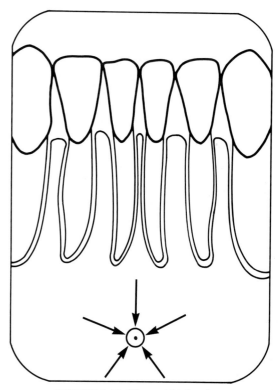

FIGURE 3–72. The genial tubercles.

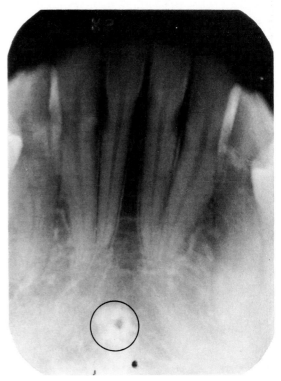

FIGURE 3–73. The genial tubercles appear as a ring-shaped radiopacity.

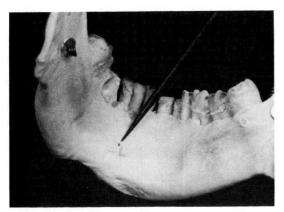

FIGURE 3–74. The lingual foramen is a small hole at the midline on the lingual surface of the mandible.

Mental Ridge

Description. The **mental ridge** is a linear prominence of cortical bone located on the external surface of the anterior portion of the mandible (Fig. 3–79). The mental ridge extends from the premolar region to the midline and slopes slightly upward.

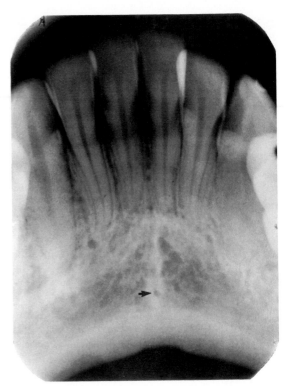

FIGURE 3–76. The lingual foramen appears as a small radiolucent dot.

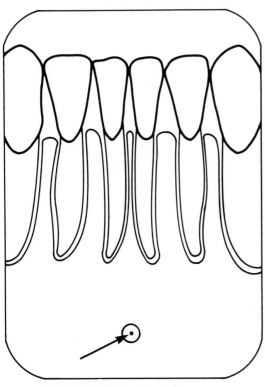

FIGURE 3–75. The lingual foramen.

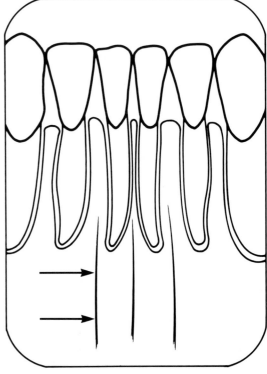

FIGURE 3–77. Nutrient canals are passageways through bone found in the mandibular anterior region.

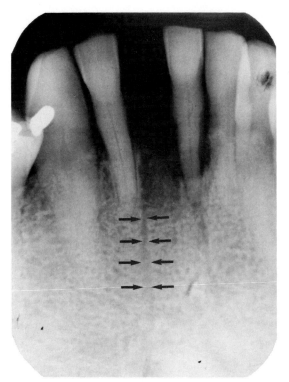

FIGURE 3–78. Nutrient canals appear as thin radiolucent lines.

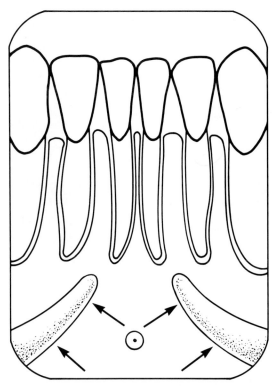

FIGURE 3–80. The mental ridge.

Radiographic Appearance. On a mandibular periapical radiograph, the mental ridge appears as a thick *radiopaque* band that extends from the premolar region to the incisor region (Figs. 3–80 and 3–81). Radiographically, the mental ridge often appears superimposed over the mandibular anterior teeth.

Mental Fossa

Description. The **mental fossa** is a scooped-out, depressed area of bone located on the external surface of the anterior mandible (Fig. 3–82).

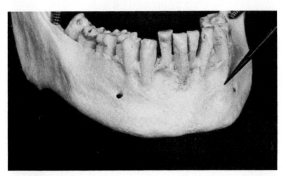

FIGURE 3–79. The mental ridge is a linear prominence of bone found on the external surface of the anterior mandible.

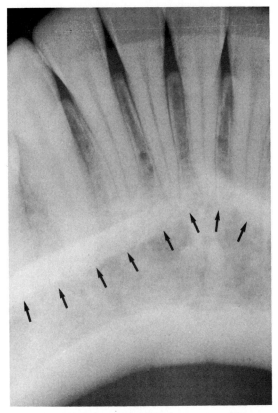

FIGURE 3–81. The mental ridge appears as a radiopaque band in the premolar and incisor region.

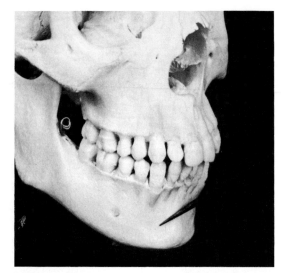

FIGURE 3–82. The mental fossa is a scooped-out or depressed area of the anterior mandible.

The mental fossa is located above the mental ridge in the mandibular incisor region.

Radiographic Appearance. On a mandibular periapical radiograph, the mental fossa appears as a *radiolucent* area above the mental ridge (Figs. 3–83 and 3–84). The radiographic appearance of the mental fossa varies and is determined by the thickness of the bone in the anterior region of the mandible.

Mental Foramen

Description. The **mental foramen** is an opening or hole in bone located on the external surface of the mandible in the region of the mandibular premolars (Fig. 3–85). Blood vessels and nerves that supply the lower lip exit through the mental foramen.

Radiographic Appearance. On a mandibular periapical radiograph, the mental foramen appears as a small ovoid or round *radiolucency* located in the apical region of the mandibular premolars (Figs. 3–86 and 3–87). The mental foramen is frequently misdiagnosed as a periapical lesion (cyst, granuloma or abscess) because of its apical location.

Mylohyoid Ridge

Description. The **mylohyoid ridge** is a linear prominence of bone located on the internal surface of the mandible (Fig. 3–88). The mylohyoid ridge extends from the molar region downward and forward toward the lower border of the mandibular symphysis. The mylohyoid ridge serves as an attachment site for a muscle of the same name.

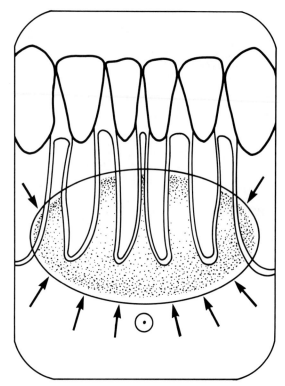

FIGURE 3–83. The mental fossa.

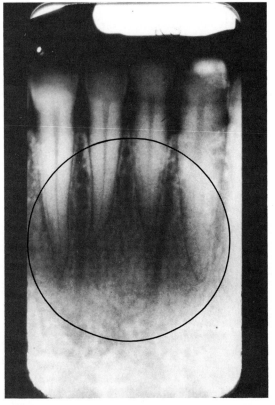

FIGURE 3–84. The mental fossa appears as a radiolucent area above the mental ridge.

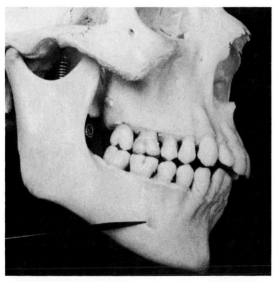

FIGURE 3–85. The mental foramen is a hole in bone located on the external surface of the mandible in the premolar area.

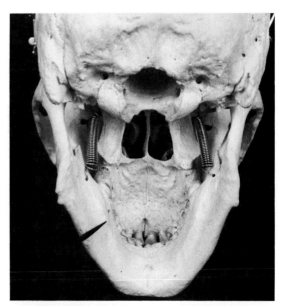

FIGURE 3–88. The mylohyoid ridge is a linear prominence of bone located on the internal surface of the mandible in the molar region.

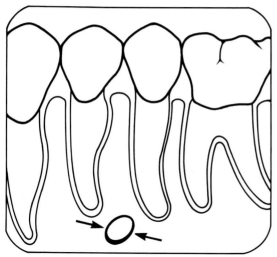

FIGURE 3–86. The mental foramen.

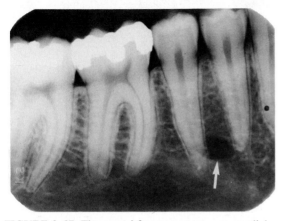

FIGURE 3–87. The mental foramen appears as a radiolucency in the mandibular premolar region.

Radiographic Appearance. On a mandibular periapical radiograph, the mylohyoid ridge appears as a dense, *radiopaque* band that extends downward and forward from the molar region (Figs. 3–89 and 3–90). The mylohyoid ridge usually appears most prominent in the molar region and may be superimposed over the roots of the mandibular teeth. The mylohyoid ridge may appear continuous with the internal oblique ridge.

Mandibular Canal

Description. The **mandibular canal** is a tube-like passageway through bone that travels the length of the mandible (Fig. 3–91). The mandibular canal extends from the mandibular foramen to the mental foramen and houses the inferior alveolar nerve and blood vessels.

Radiographic Appearance. On a mandibular periapical radiograph, the mandibular canal appears as a *radiolucent* band (Figs. 3–92 and 3–93). The mandibular canal is outlined by two thin radiopaque lines, which represent the cortical walls of the canal. The mandibular canal appears below or superimposed over the apices of the mandibular molar teeth.

Internal Oblique Ridge

Description. The **internal oblique ridge** (also known as the internal oblique line) is a linear prominence of bone located on the internal surface of the mandible that extends down-

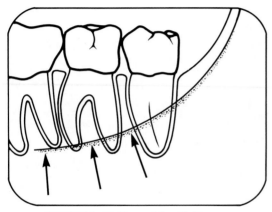

FIGURE 3–89. The mylohyoid ridge.

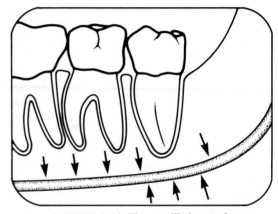

FIGURE 3–92. The mandibular canal.

ward and forward from the ramus (Fig. 3–94). The internal oblique ridge may end in the region of the mandibular third molar, or it may continue on as the mylohyoid ridge.

Radiographic Appearance. On a mandibular periapical radiograph, the internal oblique ridge appears as a *radiopaque* band that extends downward and forward from the ramus (Figs. 3–95 and 3–96). Depending upon the radiographic technique used (bisection-of-the-angle versus paralleling), the internal and external oblique ridges may be superimposed upon one another. When the ridges appear separate, the *superior* radiopaque band is the *external* oblique ridge, and the *inferior* radiopaque band is the *internal* oblique ridge.

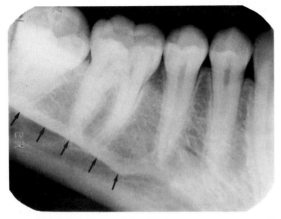

FIGURE 3–90. The mylohyoid ridge appears as a radiopaque band in the mandibular molar region.

External Oblique Ridge

Description. The **external oblique ridge** (also known as the external oblique line) is a linear prominence of bone located on the exter-

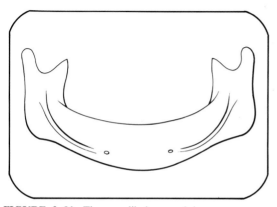

FIGURE 3–91. The mandibular canal is a passageway through bone.

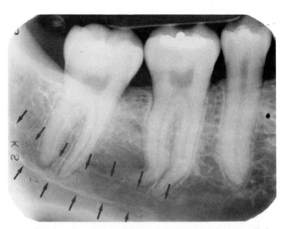

FIGURE 3–93. The mandibular canal appears as a radiolucent band outlined by two thin radiopaque lines.

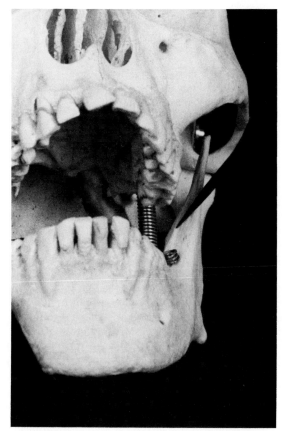

FIGURE 3–94. The internal oblique ridge is a linear prominence of bone located on the internal surface of the mandible.

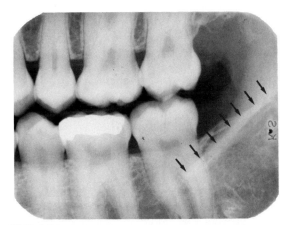

FIGURE 3–96. The internal oblique ridge appears as a radiopaque band.

of the ramus of the mandible (Figs. 3–98 and 3–99). The external oblique ridge typically ends in the mandibular third molar region.

Submandibular Fossa

Description. The **submandibular fossa** (also known as the mandibular fossa or submaxillary fossa) is a scooped-out, depressed area of bone located on the internal surface of the mandible inferior to the mylohyoid ridge (Fig. 3–100). The submandibular salivary gland is found in the submandibular fossa.

Radiographic Appearance. On a mandibular periapical radiograph, the submandibular fossa appears as a *radiolucent* area in the molar region below the mylohyoid ridge (Figs. 3–101 and 3–102). Few bony trabeculae are usually seen in the region of the submandibular fossa. On some periapical radiographs, the submandibular fossa may appear as a distinct radiolucency; in others, it may appear slightly more radiolucent than the adjacent bone.

nal surface of the body of the mandible (Fig. 3–97). The anterior border of the ramus ends in the external oblique ridge.

Radiographic Appearance. On a mandibular periapical radiograph, the external oblique ridge appears as a *radiopaque* band that extends downward and forward from the anterior border

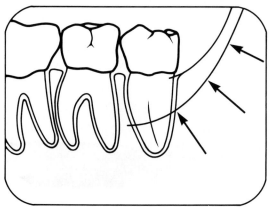

FIGURE 3–95. The internal oblique ridge.

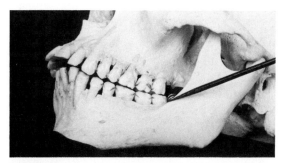

FIGURE 3–97. The external oblique ridge is a linear prominence of bone located on the external surface of the mandible.

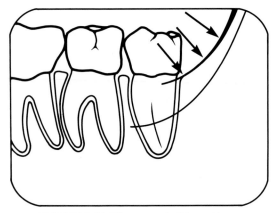

FIGURE 3–98. The external oblique ridge.

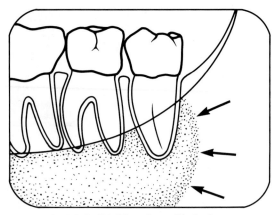

FIGURE 3–101. The submandibular fossa.

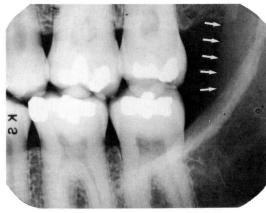

FIGURE 3–99. The external oblique ridge appears as a radiopaque band.

Coronoid Process

Description. The **coronoid process** is a marked prominence of bone found on the anterior ramus of the mandible (Fig. 3–103). The coronoid process serves as an attachment site for one of the muscles of mastication.

Radiographic Appearance. The coronoid process is *not* seen on a mandibular periapical radiograph but rather on a maxillary molar periapical film. The coronoid process appears as a triangular *radiopacity* superimposed over, or inferior to, the maxillary tuberosity region (Figs. 3–104 and 3–105).

NORMAL TOOTH ANATOMY

Tooth Structure

Tooth structures that can be viewed on dental radiographs include the following: enamel, den-

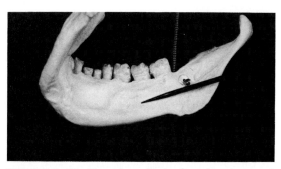

FIGURE 3–100. The submandibular fossa is a depressed area of the posterior internal surface of the mandible.

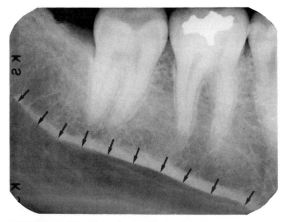

FIGURE 3–102. The submandibular fossa appears as a radiolucent area inferior to the mylohyoid ridge.

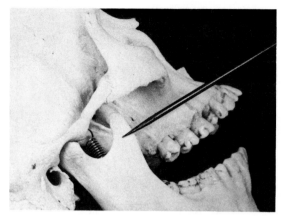

FIGURE 3–103. The coronoid process is a bony prominence on the anterior ramus of the mandible.

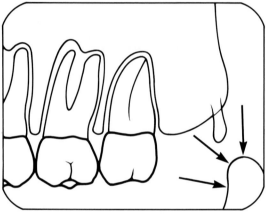

FIGURE 3–104. The coronoid process.

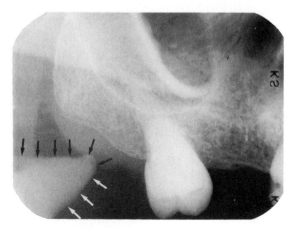

FIGURE 3–105. The coronoid process appears as a triangular-shaped radiopacity.

tin, the dentino-enamel junction and the pulp cavity (Fig. 3–106).

ENAMEL Enamel is the densest material found in the human body and appears as the outer, most *radiopaque* layer of the crown of a tooth (Fig. 3–107).

DENTIN Dentin is found beneath the enamel layer of a tooth and surrounds the pulp cavity (see Fig. 3–107). It appears *radiopaque* and comprises the majority of tooth structure. Dentin is not as radiopaque as enamel.

DENTINO-ENAMEL JUNCTION The dentino-enamel junction (DEJ) is the junction between the dentin and enamel of a tooth. The DEJ appears as a line where enamel (very radiopaque) meets the dentin (less radiopaque) (see Fig. 3–107).

PULP CAVITY The pulp cavity consists of a pulp chamber and pulp canals. It contains blood vessels, nerves and lymphatics and appears relatively *radiolucent* on a dental radiograph (Fig. 3–108). When viewed on dental radiographs, the pulp cavity is generally larger in children than in adults because it decreases in size with age due to the formation of secondary dentin. The size and shape of a pulp cavity varies with each tooth.

Supporting Structure

The alveolar process, or alveolar bone, serves as the supporting structure for the teeth of the jaws. The alveolar bone is the bone of the maxilla and mandible that supports and encases the roots of teeth (Fig. 3–109). Alveolar bone is made up of dense cortical bone and cancellous bone.

Anatomy of Alveolar Bone

The anatomic landmarks of the alveolar process include the lamina dura, alveolar crest and the periodontal ligament space (Fig. 3–110).

LAMINA DURA

Description. The **lamina dura** is the wall of the tooth socket that surrounds the root of a tooth. The lamina dura is made up of dense cortical bone.

Radiographic Appearance. On a dental radiograph, the lamina dura appears as a dense

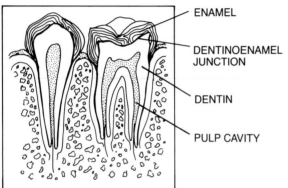

FIGURE 3–106. Tooth structures.

ENAMEL

DENTINOENAMEL JUNCTION

DENTIN

PULP CAVITY

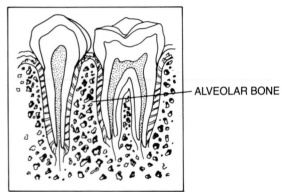

FIGURE 3–109. Alveolar bone.

ALVEOLAR BONE

radiopaque line that surrounds the root of a tooth (Fig. 3–111).

Alveolar Crest

Description. The **alveolar crest** is the most coronal portion of the alveolar bone that is found between the teeth. The alveolar crest is made up of dense cortical bone and is continuous with the lamina dura.

Radiographic Appearance. On a dental radiograph, the alveolar crest appears *radiopaque* and is typically located 1.5 to 2.0 mm below the junction of the crown and the root surfaces (the cemento-enamel junction) (Fig. 3–112).

Periodontal Ligament Space

Description. The **periodontal ligament space,** also known as "the PDL," is the space between the root of the tooth and the lamina dura. The PDL contains connective tissue fibers, blood vessels and lymphatics.

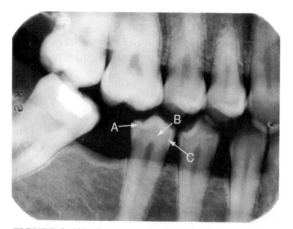

FIGURE 3–107. Tooth structures: *A*, Enamel. *B*, Dentin. *C*, Dentino-enamel junction.

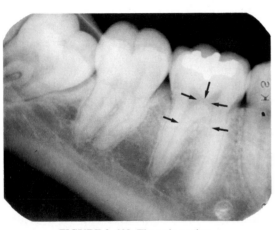

FIGURE 3–108. The pulp cavity.

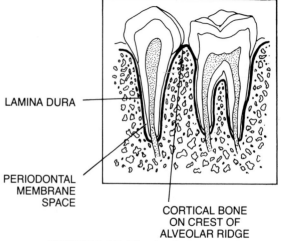

LAMINA DURA

PERIODONTAL MEMBRANE SPACE

CORTICAL BONE ON CREST OF ALVEOLAR RIDGE

FIGURE 3–110. The alveolar process.

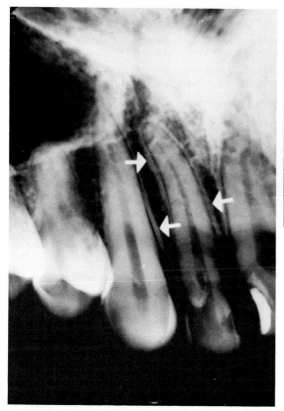

FIGURE 3-111. The lamina dura appears as a dense thin radiopaque line around the root of a tooth.

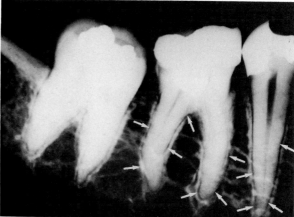

FIGURE 3-113. The periodontal ligament space appears as a thin, radiolucent line around the root of a tooth.

Shape and Density of Alveolar Bone

The alveolar bone located between the roots of the teeth varies in shape and density.

Anterior Regions. A normal alveolar crest located in the anterior region appears pointed and sharp between the teeth (Fig. 3–114). The alveolar crest appears as a dense *radiopaque* line in the anterior regions.

Radiographic Appearance. On a dental radiograph, the PDL appears as a thin *radiolucent* line around the root of a tooth. In a healthy patient, the PDL appears as a continuous radiolucent line of uniform thickness (Fig. 3–113).

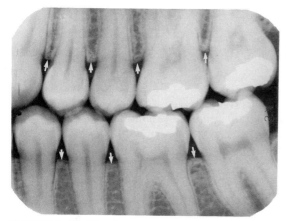

FIGURE 3-112. The alveolar crest typically appears 1.5 to 2.0 mm below the cemento-enamel junction.

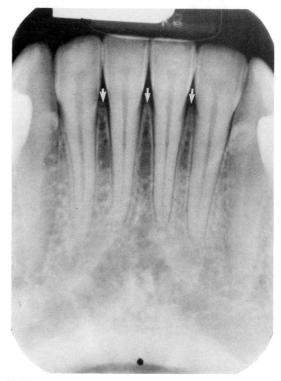

FIGURE 3-114. The anterior alveolar crest normally appears pointed and sharp.

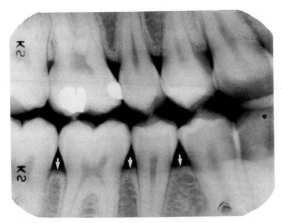

FIGURE 3–115. The posterior alveolar crest normally appears flat and smooth.

Posterior Regions. A normal alveolar crest located in the posterior region appears flat and smooth between the teeth (Fig. 3–115). The alveolar crest located in the posterior region tends to appear less dense and less *radiopaque* than the alveolar crest viewed in the anterior region.

SUMMARY

Understanding normal anatomy is important for accurate film mounting and proper interpretation of radiographs. The dental professional must have a thorough knowledge of the skull. A working knowledge of the anatomy of the maxilla, mandible and surrounding structures enables the dental professional to accurately mount dental radiographs and to distinguish maxillary periapicals from mandibular periapicals. Normal anatomic landmarks also provide cues to the proper mounting of bite-wing films.

Recognition of normal anatomic landmarks is necessary for interpretation of dental radiographs. A knowledge of normal anatomy viewed on periapical radiographs is essential before the dental professional can begin to recognize what is abnormal. One must know normal anatomy in order to recognize abnormal conditions.

Chapter 3 has reviewed the normal anatomic landmarks of the maxilla and mandible normally viewed on periapical radiographs.

Bibliography

Brand RW and Isselhard DE: Osteology of the skull. *In* Anatomy of Orofacial Structures, 4th ed., pp 117–33. St. Louis: CV Mosby, 1990.

Dental Auxiliary Education Project: Normal Radiographic Landmarks. New York: Teachers College Press, 1982.

Frommer HH: Film mounting and normal radiographic anatomy. *In* Radiology for Dental Auxiliaries, pp 232–52. St. Louis: CB Mosby, 1987.

Goaz PW and White SC: Normal radiographic anatomy. *In* Oral Radiology Principles and Interpretation, 2d ed., pp 174–99. St. Louis: CV Mosby, 1987.

Miles DA, et al: Normal anatomy and film mounting. *In* Radiographic Imaging for Dental Auxiliaries, pp 165–78. Philadelphia: WB Saunders, 1989.

QUIZ QUESTIONS

Matching

Match the following terms with the proper definitions.

__ **1.** Fossa   __ **5.** Septum

__ **2.** Canal   __ **6.** Suture

__ **3.** Foramen   __ **7.** Cortical

__ **4.** Sinus   __ **8.** Cancellous

A. Hole or opening in bone
B. Broad shallow depression in bone
C. Cavity, recess or hollow space in bone
D. Passageway through bone

E. Sponge-like bone
F. Bony partition that separates two spaces
G. Immovable joint found between bones
H. Hard or compact bone

"What Can This Be?"

1. Identify the normal anatomical feature in Figure 3–116.

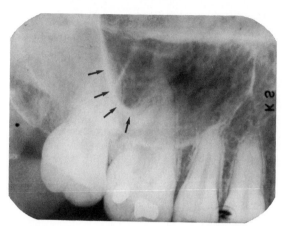

FIGURE 3–116.

2. Identify the normal anatomical feature in Figure 3–117.

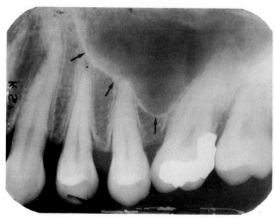

FIGURE 3–117.

3. Identify the normal anatomical feature in Figure 3–118.

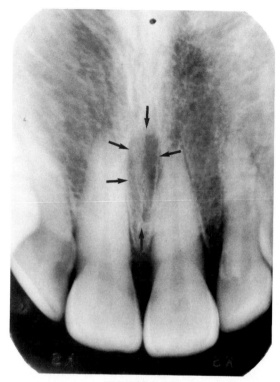

FIGURE 3–118.

4. Identify the normal anatomical feature in Figure 3–119.

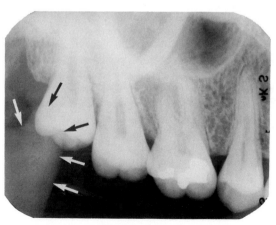

FIGURE 3–119.

5. Identify the normal anatomical feature in Figure 3–120.

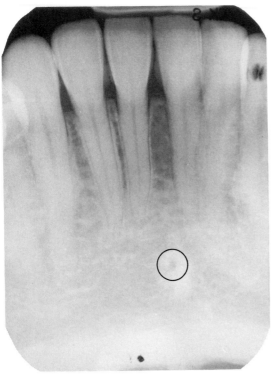

FIGURE 3–120.

6. Identify the normal anatomical feature in Figure 3–121.

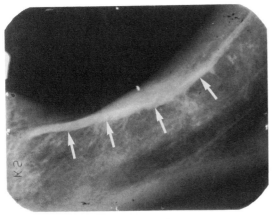

FIGURE 3–121.

7. Identify the normal anatomical feature in Figure 3–122.

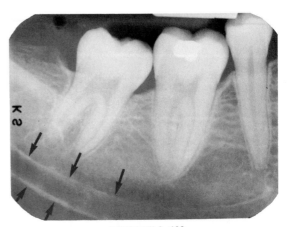

FIGURE 3–122.

8. Identify the normal anatomical feature in Figure 3–123.

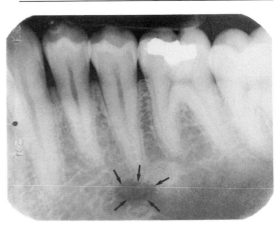

FIGURE 3–123.

Normal Anatomy (Panoramic Films)

Objectives   After completion of this chapter, the student will be able to:

▶ Identify and describe the bony landmarks of the maxilla and surrounding structures as viewed on the panoramic radiograph.

▶ Identify and describe the bony landmarks of the mandible and surrounding structures as viewed on the panoramic radiograph.

▶ Identify air space images as viewed on the panoramic radiograph.

▶ Identify soft tissue images as viewed on the panoramic radiograph.

▶ Identify artifacts as viewed on the panoramic radiograph.

▶ Identify positioning errors viewed on a panoramic radiograph.

▶ Discuss the causes of positioning errors viewed on panoramic radiographs.

▶ Discuss the measures necessary to correct positioning errors viewed on panoramic radiographs.

Key Words

Ala-tragus line
Angle of the mandible
Anterior nasal spine
Articular eminence
Coronoid notch
Coronoid process
External auditory meatus
External oblique ridge
Focal trough
Frankfort plane
Genial tubercles
Ghost image
Glenoid fossa
Glossopharyngeal air space
Hamulus

Hard palate
Hyoid bone
Incisive canal
Inferior border of the mandible
Infraorbital foramen
Internal oblique ridge
Lateral pterygoid plate
Lingual foramen
Lingula
Mandibular canal
Mandibular condyle
Mandibular foramen
Mastoid process
Maxillary sinus
Maxillary tuberosity

Mental foramen
Mental fossa
Mental ridge
Midsagittal plane
Mylohyoid ridge
Nasal cavity
Nasal septum
Nasopharyngeal air space
Orbit
Palatoglossal air space
Panoramic
Styloid process
Submandibular shadow
Zygoma
Zygomatic process

A panoramic radiograph allows the dental professional to view a large area of the mandible and maxilla on a single film. Just as dental professionals must be able to recognize normal anatomic landmarks on periapical films, they must also be able to recognize normal anatomic structures viewed on panoramic radiographs. The recognition of radiographic landmarks enables dental professionals to accurately interpret panoramic films. Without a working knowledge of anatomy, they may mistake normal anatomic structures for pathologic conditions.

In order to interpret the panoramic radiograph and identify normal anatomic landmarks, dental professionals must have a thorough knowledge of the anatomy of maxilla and mandible. Each normal anatomic landmark seen on a panoramic radiograph corresponds to what is seen on the human skull. If dental professionals are familiar with the anatomy of the human skull, they can identify the normal anatomy viewed on a panoramic radiograph.

In addition to the normal anatomic landmarks, air space images, soft tissue images and artifacts are also presented in Chapter 4. Common panoramic positioning errors are also discussed.

NORMAL ANATOMIC LANDMARKS

Bony Landmarks of the Maxilla and Surrounding Structures

As previously described, the maxilla forms the floor of the orbit of the eyes, the sides and floor of the nasal cavity and the hard palate. The lower border of the maxilla supports the maxillary teeth. This portion of the chapter reviews the bony landmarks of the maxilla and surrounding structures that can be viewed on panoramic radiographs.

Each of the following bony landmarks of the maxilla and surrounding structures can be found labelled on Figure 4–1.

Mastoid Process

Description. The **mastoid process** is a marked prominence of bone located posterior and inferior to the temporomandibular joint (TMJ). The mastoid process is part of the temporal bone.

Radiographic Appearance. On a panoramic radiograph, the mastoid process appears as a rounded *radiopacity* located posterior and inferior to the TMJ area. The mastoid process is *not* seen on periapical radiographs.

Styloid Process

Description. The **styloid process** is a long, pointed and sharp projection of bone that extends downward from the inferior surface of the temporal bone. The styloid process is located anterior to the mastoid process.

Radiographic Appearance. On a panoramic radiograph, the styloid process appears as a long *radiopaque* spine that extends from the temporal bone anterior to the mastoid process. The styloid process is *not* seen on periapical radiographs.

External Auditory Meatus

Description. The **external auditory meatus** (also known as the external acoustic meatus) is a hole or opening in the temporal bone located superior and anterior to the mastoid process.

Radiographic Appearance. On a panoramic radiograph, the external auditory meatus appears as a round to ovoid *radiolucency* anterior and superior to the mastoid process. The external auditory meatus is *not* seen on periapical radiographs.

Glenoid Fossa

Description. The **glenoid fossa** (also known as the mandibular fossa) is a concave, depressed area of the temporal bone. The mandibular condyle rests in the glenoid fossa. The glenoid fossa is located anterior to the mastoid process and the external auditory meatus.

Radiographic Appearance. On a panoramic radiograph, the glenoid fossa appears as a concave *radiopacity* superior to the mandibular condyle. The glenoid fossa is *not* seen on periapical radiographs.

Articular Eminence

Description. The **articular eminence** (also known as the articular tubercle) is a rounded projection of the temporal bone located anterior to the glenoid fossa.

Radiographic Appearance. On a panoramic radiograph, the articular eminence appears as a rounded *radiopaque* projection of bone located anterior to the glenoid fossa. The

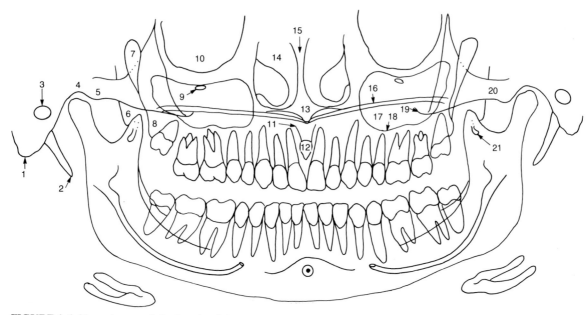

FIGURE 4–1. Normal anatomic landmarks of the maxilla and surrounding structures: *1*, mastoid process; *2*, styloid process; *3*, external auditory meatus; *4*, glenoid fossa; *5*, articular eminence; *6*, lateral pterygoid plate; *7*, pterygomaxillary fissure; *8*, maxillary tuberosity; *9*, infraorbital foramen; *10*, orbit; *11*, incisive canal; *12*, incisive foramen; *13*, anterior nasal spine; *14*, nasal cavity and conchae; *15*, nasal septum; *16*, hard palate; *17*, maxillary sinus; *18*, floor of maxillary sinus; *19*, zygomatic process of maxilla; *20*, zygomatic arch; *21*, hamulus. (Modified from Dental Auxiliary Education Projects: Normal Radiographic Landmarks. New York: Teachers College Press, 1982.)

articular eminence is *not* seen on periapical radiographs.

Lateral Pterygoid Plate

Description. The **lateral pterygoid plate** is a wing-shaped bony projection of the sphenoid bone located distal to the maxillary tuberosity region.

Radiographic Appearance. On a panoramic radiograph, the lateral pterygoid plate appears as a *radiopaque* projection of bone distal to the maxillary tuberosity region. The lateral pterygoid plate is *not* seen on periapical radiographs.

Pterygomaxillary Fissure

Description. The **pterygomaxillary fissure** is a narrow space or cleft that separates the lateral pterygoid plate and the maxilla.

Radiographic Appearance. On a panoramic radiograph, the pterygomaxillary fissure appears as a *radiolucent* area between the lateral pterygoid plate and the maxilla. The zygoma is often superimposed over this region and obscures the pterygomaxillary fissure. The pterygomaxillary fissure is *not* seen on periapical radiographs.

Maxillary Tuberosity

Description. The **maxillary tuberosity** is a rounded prominence of bone that extends posterior to the third molar region.

Radiographic Appearance. On a panoramic radiograph, the maxillary tuberosity appears as a *radiopaque* bulge distal to the third molar region.

Infraorbital Foramen

Description. The **infraorbital foramen** is a hole or opening in bone found inferior to the border of the orbit.

Radiographic Appearance. On a panoramic radiograph, the infraorbital foramen appears as a round or ovoid *radiolucency* inferior to the orbit. The infraorbital foramen may be superimposed over the maxillary sinus. The infraorbital foramen is *not* seen on periapical radiographs.

Orbit

Description. The **orbit** is the bony cavity that contains the eyeball.

Radiographic Appearance. On a panoramic radiograph, the orbit appears as a round *radiolucent* compartment with radiopaque borders located superior to the maxillary sinuses. On most panoramic radiographs, only the inferior border of the orbit is visible and appears as a radiopaque line.

Incisive Canal

Description. The **incisive canal** (also known as the nasopalatine canal) is a passageway through bone that extends from the superior foramina of the incisive canal (located on the floor of the nasal cavity) to the incisive foramen (located on the anterior hard palate).

Radiographic Appearance. On a panoramic radiograph, the incisive canal appears as a tube-like *radiolucent* area with radiopaque borders. The incisive canal is located between the maxillary central incisors.

Incisive Foramen

Description. The **incisive foramen** (also known as the nasopalatine foramen) is an opening or hole in bone that is located at the midline of the anterior portion of the hard palate directly posterior to the maxillary central incisors.

Radiographic Appearance. On a panoramic radiograph, the incisive foramen appears as a small ovoid or round *radiolucency* located between the roots of the maxillary central incisors.

Anterior Nasal Spine

Description. The **anterior nasal spine** is a sharp bony projection of the maxilla located at the anterior and inferior portion of the nasal cavity.

Radiographic Appearance. On a panoramic radiograph, the anterior nasal spine appears as a V-shaped *radiopaque* area located at the intersection of the floor of the nasal cavity and the nasal septum.

Nasal Cavity

Description. The **nasal cavity** (also known as the nasal fossa) is a pear-shaped compartment of bone located superior to the maxilla.

Radiographic Appearance. On a panoramic radiograph, the nasal cavity appears as a large *radiolucent* area above the maxillary incisors.

Nasal Septum

Description. The **nasal septum** is a vertical bony wall or partition that divides the nasal cavity into the right and left nasal fossae.

Radiographic Appearance. On a panoramic radiograph, the nasal septum appears as a vertical *radiopaque* partition that divides the nasal cavity.

Hard Palate

Description. The **hard palate** is the bony wall that separates the nasal cavity from the oral cavity.

Radiographic Appearance. On a panoramic radiograph, the hard palate appears as a horizontal *radiopaque* band superior to the apices of the maxillary teeth.

Maxillary Sinus and Floor of Maxillary Sinus

Description. The **maxillary sinuses** are paired cavities or compartments of bone located within the maxilla and are located above the maxillary premolar and molar teeth.

Radiographic Appearance. On a panoramic radiograph, the maxillary sinuses appear as paired *radiolucent* areas located above the apices of the maxillary premolars and molars. The floor of the maxillary sinus is composed of dense cortical bone and appears as a radiopaque line.

Zygomatic Process of the Maxilla

Description. The **zygomatic process of the maxilla** is a bony projection of the maxilla that articulates with the zygoma or malar (cheek) bone.

Radiographic Appearance. On a panoramic radiograph, the zygomatic process of the maxilla appears as a J- or U-shaped *radiopacity* located superior to the maxillary first molar region.

Zygoma

Description. The **zygoma** (also known as the malar or zygomatic bone) is the cheek bone and articulates with the zygomatic process of the maxilla.

Radiographic Appearance. On a panoramic radiograph, the zygoma appears as a *radiopaque* band that extends posteriorly from the zygomatic process of the maxilla.

Hamulus

Description. The **hamulus** (also known as the hamular process) is a small hook-like projection of bone that extends from the medial pterygoid plate of the sphenoid bone. The hamulus is located posterior to the maxillary tuberosity region.

Radiographic Appearance. On a panoramic radiograph, the hamulus appears as a *radiopaque* hook-like projection posterior to the maxillary tuberosity area.

Figures 4–2, 4–3, and 4–4 illustrate the normal anatomic landmarks of the maxilla and surrounding structures that can be viewed on a panoramic radiograph.

Bony Landmarks of the Mandible and Surrounding Structures

This portion of Chapter 4 reviews the bony landmarks of the mandible and surrounding structures that can be viewed on a panoramic radiograph. Each of the following bony landmarks of the mandible and surrounding structures can be found labeled on Figure 4–5.

Mandibular Condyle

Description. The **mandibular condyle** is a rounded projection of bone extending from the posterior superior border of the ramus of the mandible. The mandibular condyle articulates with the glenoid fossa of the temporal bone.

Radiographic Appearance. On a panoramic radiograph, the mandibular condyle appears as a bony rounded *radiopaque* projection extending from the posterior border of the ramus of the mandible. The mandibular condyle is *not* seen on periapical radiographs.

Coronoid Notch

Description. The **coronoid notch** is a scooped-out concavity of bone located distal to the coronoid process of the mandible.

Radiographic Appearance. On a panoramic radiograph, the coronoid notch appears as a *radiopaque* concavity located distal to the coronoid process on the superior border of the ramus. The coronoid notch is *not* seen on periapical radiographs.

Coronoid Process

Description. The **coronoid process** is a marked prominence of bone found on the anterior superior ramus of the mandible.

Radiographic Appearance. On a panoramic radiograph, the coronoid process appears as a triangular *radiopacity* posterior to the maxillary tuberosity region.

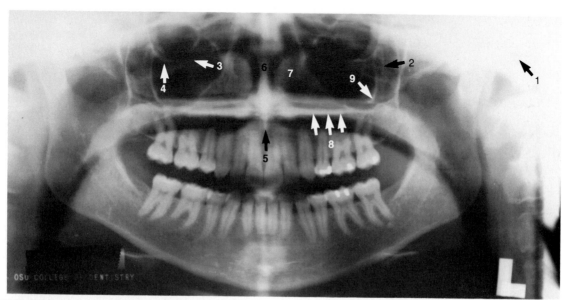

FIGURE 4–2. Normal anatomic landmarks of the maxilla and surrounding structures seen on panoramic films: *1*, external auditory meatus; *2*, pterygomaxillary fissure; *3*, infraorbital foramen; *4*, orbit; *5*, anterior nasal spine; *6*, nasal septum; *7*, nasal conchae; *8*, hard palate; *9*, zygomatic process of the maxilla.

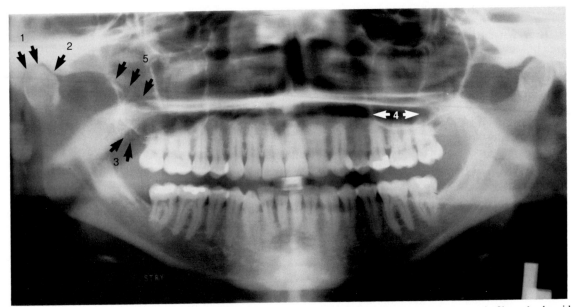

FIGURE 4–3. Normal anatomic landmarks of the maxilla and surrounding structures seen on panoramic films: *1*, glenoid fossa; *2*, articular eminence; *3*, maxillary tuberosity; *4*, maxillary sinus; *5*, zygoma.

Mandibular Foramen

Description. The **mandibular foramen** is a round or ovoid hole in bone on the lingual aspect of the ramus of the mandible.

Radiographic Appearance. On a panoramic radiograph, the mandibular foramen appears as a round or ovoid *radiolucency* centered within the ramus of the mandible. The mandibular foramen is *not* seen on periapical radiographs.

Lingula

Description. The **lingula** is a small tongue-shaped projection of bone seen adjacent to the mandibular foramen.

Radiographic Appearance. On a panoramic radiograph, the lingula appears as an indistinct *radiopacity* anterior to the mandibular foramen. The lingula is *not* seen on periapical radiographs.

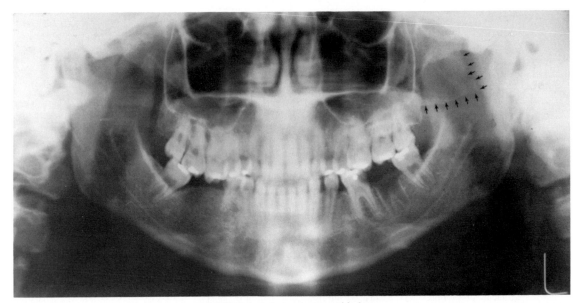

FIGURE 4–4. Lateral pterygoid plate.

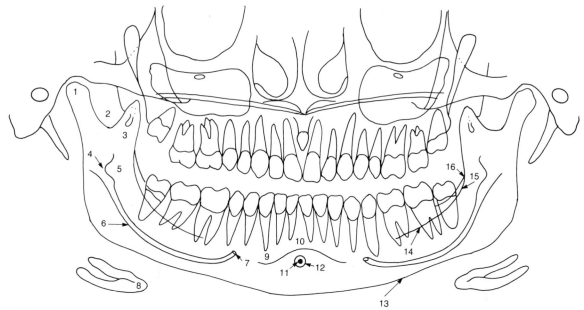

FIGURE 4–5. Normal anatomic landmarks of the mandible and surrounding structures: *1*, condyle; *2*, coronoid notch; *3*, coronoid process; *4*, mandibular foramen; *5*, lingula; *6*, mandibular canal; *7*, mental foramen; *8*, hyoid bone; *9*, mental ridge; *10*, mental fossa; *11*, lingual foramen; *12*, genial tubercles; *13*, inferior border of mandible; *14*, mylohyoid ridge; *15*, internal oblique ridge; *16*, external oblique ridge. (Modified from Dental Auxiliary Education Project: Normal Radiographic Landmarks. New York: Teachers College Press, 1982.)

Mandibular Canal

Description. The **mandibular canal** is a tube-like passageway through bone that travels the length of the mandible. The mandibular canal extends from the mandibular foramen to the mental foramen and houses the inferior alveolar nerve and blood vessels.

Radiographic Appearance. On a panoramic radiograph, the mandibular canal appears as a *radiolucent* band outlined by two thin radiopaque lines representing the cortical walls of the canal.

Mental Foramen

Description. The **mental foramen** is an opening or hole in bone located on the external surface of the mandible in the region of the mandibular premolars.

Radiographic Appearance. On a panoramic radiograph, the mental foramen appears as a small ovoid or round *radiolucency* located in the apical region of the mandibular premolars.

Hyoid

Description. The **hyoid** is a horseshoe-shaped bone located at the base of the tongue just below the thyroid cartilage.

Radiographic Appearance. On a panoramic radiograph, the hyoid appears as a U-shaped *radiopacity* located inferior to the ramus of the mandible. The hyoid bone is *not* seen in periapical radiographs.

Mental Ridge

Description. The **mental ridge** is a linear prominence of cortical bone located on the external surface of the anterior portion of the mandible that extends from the premolar region to the midline.

Radiographic Appearance. On a panoramic radiograph, the mental ridge appears as a thick *radiopaque* band that extends from the mandibular premolar region to the incisor region.

Mental Fossa

Description. The **mental fossa** is a scooped-out depressed area of bone located on the external surface of the anterior mandible above the mental ridge in the mandibular incisor region.

Radiographic Appearance. On a panoramic radiograph, the mental fossa appears as a *radiolucent* area above the mental ridge.

Lingual Foramen

Description. The **lingual foramen** is a tiny opening or hole in bone located on the internal surface of the mandible near the midline.

Radiographic Appearance. On a panoramic radiograph, the lingual foramen appears as a small *radiolucent* dot located inferior to the apices of the mandibular incisors.

Genial Tubercles

Description. The **genial tubercles** are tiny bumps of bone located on the lingual aspect of the mandible.

Radiographic Appearance. On a panoramic radiograph, the genial tubercles appear as a ring-shaped *radiopacity* surrounding the lingual foramen.

Inferior Border of the Mandible

Description. The **inferior border of the mandible** is a linear prominence of cortical bone that defines the lower border of the mandible.

Radiographic Appearance. On a panoramic radiograph, the inferior border of the mandible appears as a dense *radiopaque* band that outlines the lower border of the mandible.

Mylohyoid Ridge

Description. The **mylohyoid ridge** is a linear prominence of bone located on the internal surface of the mandible that extends from the molar region downward and forward toward the lower border of the mandibular symphysis.

Radiographic Appearance. On a panoramic radiograph, the mylohyoid ridge appears as a dense *radiopaque* band that extends downward and forward from the molar region.

Internal Oblique Ridge

Description. The **internal oblique ridge** is a linear prominence of bone located on the internal surface of the mandible that extends downward and forward from the ramus.

Radiographic Appearance. On a panoramic radiograph, the internal oblique ridge appears as a *radiopaque* band that extends downward and forward from the ramus.

External Oblique Ridge

Description. The **external oblique ridge** is a linear prominence of bone located on the external surface of the body of the mandible.

Radiographic Appearance. On a panoramic radiograph, the external oblique ridge appears as a *radiopaque* band that extends downward and forward from the anterior border of the ramus of the mandible.

Angle of the Mandible

Description. The **angle of the mandible** is the area of the mandible where the body meets the ramus.

Radiographic Appearance. On a panoramic radiograph, the angle of the mandible appears as a *radiopaque* bony structure where the ramus joins the body of the mandible.

Figures 4–6, 4–7 and 4–8 illustrate the normal anatomic landmarks of the mandible and surrounding structures that can be viewed on a panoramic radiograph.

AIR SPACE IMAGES SEEN ON PANORAMIC RADIOGRAPHS

This portion of Chapter 4 reviews the air space images that can be viewed on a panoramic radiograph. Each of the following air space images can be found labeled on Figure 4–9.

Palatoglossal Air Space

Description. The **palatoglossal air space** refers to the space found between the palate (*palato*) and tongue (*glossal*).

Radiographic Appearance. On a panoramic radiograph, the palatoglossal air space appears as a horizontal *radiolucent* band located above the apices of the maxillary teeth.

Nasopharyngeal Air Space

Description. The **nasopharyngeal air space** refers to the portion of the pharynx (*pharyngeal*) located posterior to the nasal cavity (*naso*).

Radiographic Appearance. On a panoramic radiograph, the nasopharyngeal air space appears as a diagonal *radiolucency* located superior to the radiopaque shadow of the soft palate and uvula.

Glossopharyngeal Air Space

Description. The **glossopharyngeal air space** refers to the portion of the pharynx (*pharyngeal*) located posterior to the tongue (*glosso*) and oral cavity.

Radiographic Appearance. On a panoramic radiograph, the glossopharyngeal air space appears as a vertical *radiolucent* band superimposed over the ramus of the mandible. The glossopharyngeal air space is continuous with the nasopharyngeal air space superiorly and the palatoglossal air space inferiorly.

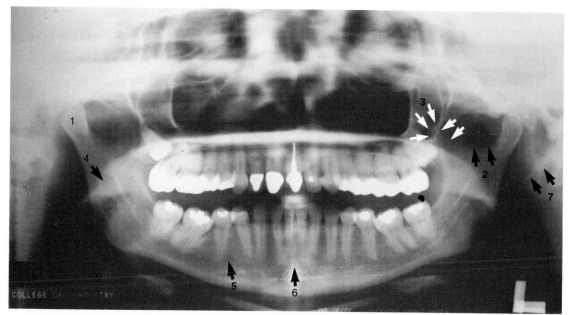

FIGURE 4–6. Normal anatomic landmarks of the mandible and surrounding structures seen on panoramic films: *1*, condyle; *2*, coronoid notch; *3*, coronoid process; *4*, mandibular foramen; *5*, mental foramen; *6*, genial tubercles; *7*, styloid process.

Figure 4–10 illustrates the air space images that can be viewed on a panoramic radiograph.

SOFT TISSUE IMAGES SEEN ON PANORAMIC RADIOGRAPHS

This portion of Chapter 4 reviews the soft tissue images that can be viewed on a panoramic radio-graph. Each of the following soft tissue images can be found labeled on Figure 4–11.

Tongue

Description. The **tongue** is a mobile muscular organ found attached to the floor of the mouth.

Radiographic Appearance. On a panoramic radiograph, the tongue appears as a *radiopaque* area superimposed over the maxillary posterior teeth.

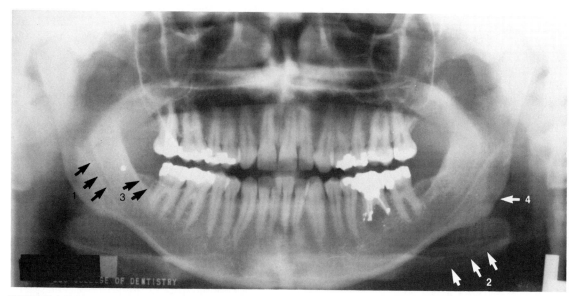

FIGURE 4–7. Normal anatomic landmarks of the mandible and surrounding structures seen on panoramic films: *1*, mandibular canal; *2*, hyoid; *3*, internal oblique ridge; *4*, angle of the mandible.

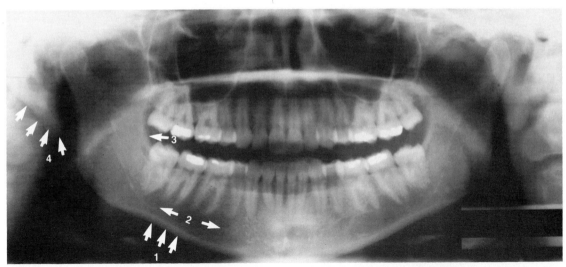

FIGURE 4–8. Normal anatomic landmarks of the mandible and surrounding structures as seen on panoramic films: *1*, inferior border of the mandible; *2*, submandibular fossa; *3*, external oblique ridge; *4*, soft tissue of the ear.

Soft Palate and Uvula

Description. The **soft palate and uvula** is a muscular curtain that separates the oral cavity from the nasal cavity.

Radiographic Appearance. On a panoramic radiograph, the soft palate and uvula appears as a diagonal *radiopacity* projecting posteriorly and inferiorly from the maxillary tuberosity region.

Lipline

Description. The **lipline** is formed by the position of the patient's lips.

Radiographic Appearance. On a panoramic radiograph, the lipline is seen in the region of the anterior teeth. The areas of the teeth not covered by the lips appear more *radiolucent*; the areas covered by the lips appear more *radiopaque*.

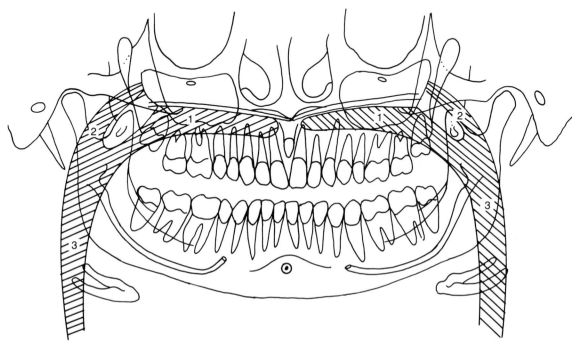

FIGURE 4–9. Air space images seen on panoramic films: *1*, palatoglossal air space; *2*, nasopharyngeal air space; *3*, glossopharyngeal air space. (Modified from Dental Auxiliary Education Project: Normal Radiographic Landmarks. New York: Teachers College Press, 1982.)

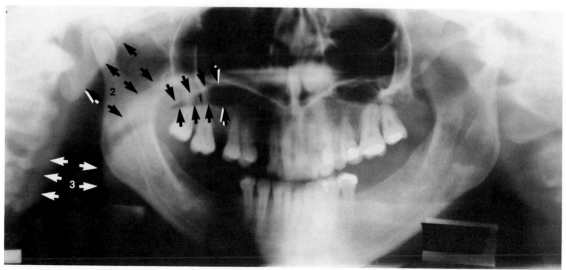

FIGURE 4–10. Air space images seen on panoramic films: *1*, palatoglossal air space; *2*, nasopharyngeal air space; *3*, glossopharyngeal air space.

Ear

Radiographic Appearance. On a panoramic radiograph, the **ear** appears as a *radiopaque* shadow that projects anteriorly and inferiorly from the mastoid process. The ear is found superimposed over the styloid process.

Figure 4–12 shows the soft tissue images that can be viewed on a panoramic radiograph.

ARTIFACTS SEEN ON PANORAMIC RADIOGRAPHS

This portion of Chapter 4 reviews artifacts that can be viewed on a panoramic radiograph. Each of the following artifacts can be found labeled on Figure 4–13.

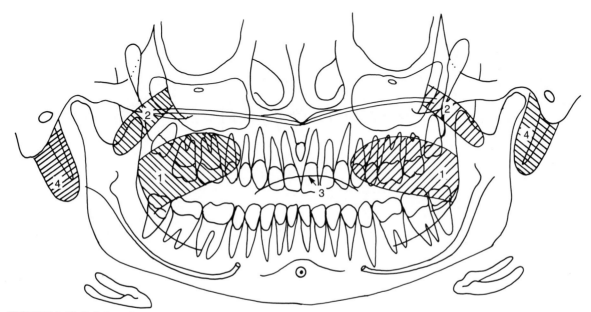

FIGURE 4–11. Soft tissue images seen on panoramic films: *1*, tongue; *2*, soft palate and uvula; *3*, lipline; *4*, ear. (Modified from Dental Auxiliary Education Project: Normal Radiographic Landmarks. New York: Teachers College Press, 1982.)

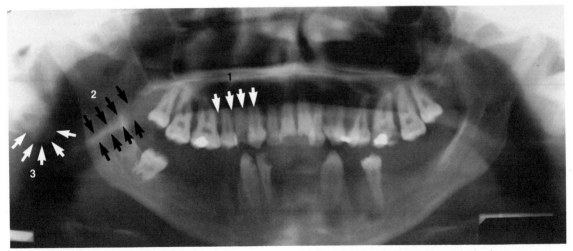

FIGURE 4–12. Soft tissue images seen on panoramic films: *1*, tongue; *2*, soft palate and uvula; *3*, ear.

Vertebral Column

Radiographic Appearance. On a panoramic radiograph, the vertebral column appears as a vertical *radiopaque* band lateral to the image of the jaws. Depending on the panoramic machine used, the vertebral column may appear superimposed over the midline in the maxillary region.

Submandibular Shadow

Radiographic Appearance. On a panoramic radiograph, the submandibular shadow is an area of increased *radiolucency* seen apical to the mandibular posterior teeth. This area of increased radiolucency results from the absence of superimposed structures inferior to the mandibular posterior teeth.

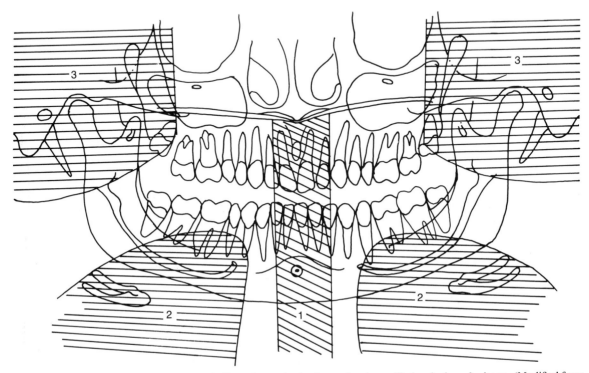

FIGURE 4–13. Artifacts seen on panoramic films: *1*, vertebral column; *2*, submandibular shadow; *3*, ghosts. (Modified from Dental Auxiliary Education Project: Normal Radiographic Landmarks. New York: Teachers College Press, 1982.)

Ghosts

Description. Ghosts (also referred to as phantoms) are produced when an area of increased density is penetrated twice by the x-ray beam. A secondary image, or ghost, is produced in addition to the primary image of the structure being radiographed.

Radiographic Appearance. On a panoramic radiograph, a ghost appears as a *radiopaque* structure. A ghost is located on the opposite side from the primary image and higher than the primary image. A ghost appears magnified, indistinct and laterally distorted.

Figures 4–14, 4–15 and 4–16 illustrate the artifact images that can be viewed on a panoramic radiograph.

POSITIONING ERRORS SEEN ON PANORAMIC RADIOGRAPHS

The panoramic film allows the dental professional to view a single image of the facial structures, including the maxillary and mandibular arches, the maxillary sinuses, the lower border of the orbits, the temporomandibular joints and adjoining anatomic structures. The panoramic radiograph is a valuable diagnostic tool that enables the practitioner to identify many conditions and diseases which may otherwise go undetected.

Panoramic radiographs, as with all dental radiographs, must be properly prescribed, exposed and processed to minimize the biological effects of ionizing radiation. In order to produce diagnostic panoramic radiographs and minimize patient exposure, mistakes must be avoided. Some of the more common errors seen in panoramic radiography include mistakes in patient preparation and patient positioning.

Patient Preparation Errors

Proper patient preparation is critical in obtaining a diagnostic panoramic film. Two of the more common patient preparation errors include the production of ghost images and the lead apron artifact.

Ghost Images

Problem

Before exposing a panoramic film, all metallic or radiodense objects must be removed from the patient's head and neck region. Eyeglasses, earrings, necklaces, hairpins, removable partial dentures, complete dentures, orthodontic retainers, hearing aids and patient napkin chains must be removed. Failure to remove any of these items results in a radiopacity, or ghost image, that obscures information concerning the area being radiographed.

A ghost image is formed when a metallic or radiodense object is located between the x-ray source and the structures being radiographed. A

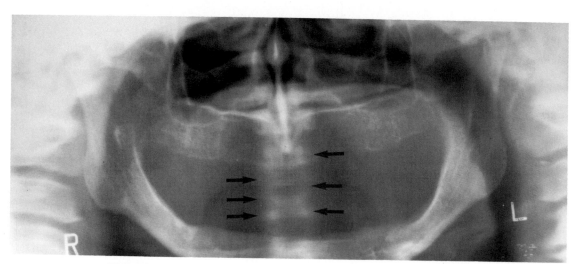

FIGURE 4–14. Cervical spine seen superimposed over the midline of the film.

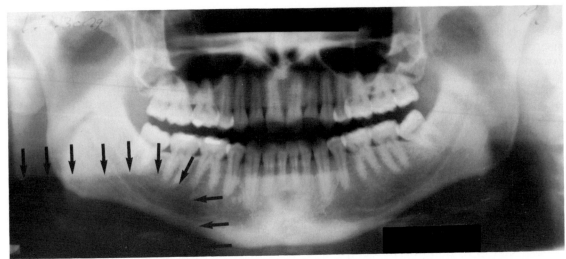

FIGURE 4–15. Submandibular shadow artifact.

ghost image essentially looks like its real counterpart but appears larger, on the opposite side and higher than its actual counterpart. For example, a ghost image of a hoop earring appears as a radiopacity that is *larger,* on the *opposite* side and *higher* than the real hoop earring. In addition, the ghost image of the hoop earring appears *blurred* or smeared in both a horizontal and vertical direction (Fig. 4–17). Ghost images interfere with the interpretation of panoramic radiographs by obscuring information.

Solution

To prevent ghost images, always look for obvious metallic objects, such as jewelry and intraoral appliances. Ask the patient to remove all

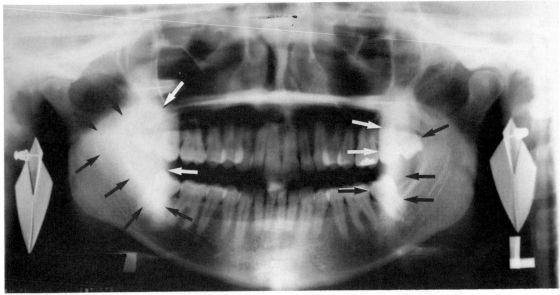

FIGURE 4–16. Large metallic earrings produce large ghost images.

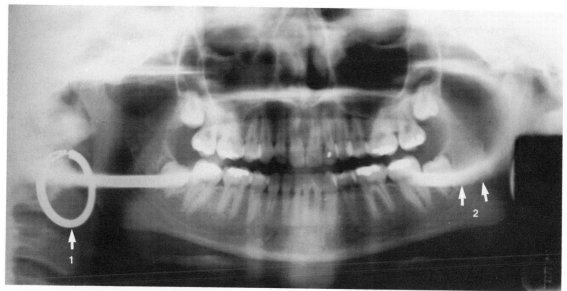

FIGURE 4–17. Large hoop earrings (*1*) and ghost images (*2*). The ghost image of the earring appears on the opposite side of the film and is enlarged and laterally distorted.

jewelry and intraoral appliances *before* positioning the patient for a panoramic film. Observe your patient carefully. Less obvious metallic objects such as hearing aids, nose jewelry, or hairpins (perhaps securing a wig) must also be removed before exposing the panoramic film.

Lead Apron Artifact

Problem

In order to limit the amount of scatter radiation that reaches the reproductive organs of the patient, the use of a lead apron *without* a thyroid collar is recommended during panoramic radiography. A thyroid collar or cervical shield is not recommended for panoramic radiography because it produces a large radiopacity over the mandibular area of the radiograph. The operator must be aware of lead apron placement. A lead apron placed too high on the neck of the patient produces a radiopaque cone-shaped artifact on the resultant film (Fig. 4–18).

Solution

The radiopaque artifact from a misplaced lead apron may mask diagnostic information vital to the health of the patient. To avoid this error, the operator should place the lead apron *without* a thyroid collar on the patient taking special care not to place the apron too high around the patient's neck.

Patient Positioning Errors

Patient positioning is of critical importance when preparing to expose a panoramic film. Since the panoramic image does not resolve the fine anatomic detail seen on intraoral radiographs, even the smallest positioning error can create a distorted image. Careful positioning of the patient's head can reduce panoramic film errors.

Positioning Tips

- The panoramic machine may elicit some apprehension on the part of the patient. A brief explanation concerning the procedure should answer any questions and reassure the patient.
- The patient should be instructed to sit or stand "as tall as possible" with the back straight and erect.
- The patient's chin must be positioned on the chin rest.
- The operator should next instruct the patient to do the following: bite on the plastic bite block, place their front teeth in an end-to-end position in the groove found on the bite block (Fig. 4–19) and close their lips on the bite block. In machines not equipped with a bite block, a cotton roll can be used to separate the maxillary and mandibular incisors and prevent vertical overlap.

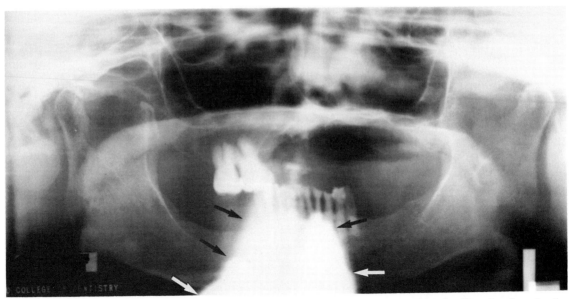

FIGURE 4–18. On a panoramic radiograph, a lead apron artifact appears as a large cone-shaped radiopacity obscuring the mandible.

- The patient's **Frankfort plane** (the imaginary plane that intersects the orbital rim of the eyes and the ear openings) must be parallel with the floor, and the **ala-tragus line** should be tipped approximately 5 degrees downward (Fig. 4–20).
- The operator must adjust the anterior guide bar to firmly support the patient's forehead.
- The patient's **midsagittal plane** must be positioned perpendicular to the floor. The operator should make certain that the patient's head is not tipped or tilted.
- The patient's head should be centered by adjusting the side guide bars so they firmly contact the sides of the patient's head.
- The operator should instruct the patient to swallow and place their tongue on the roof of the mouth.
- The operator should remind the patient to remain very still during the exposure.

Proper patient positioning is critical in obtaining a diagnostic panoramic film. Some of the more common patient positioning errors include the incorrect positioning of the head, lips, tongue, chin and teeth.

Lip and Tongue Position

Problem

The correct position of the patient's lips and tongue adds to the diagnostic quality of the panoramic film. If the patient's lips are not closed on the bite block during the exposure cycle of the panoramic machine, a dark radiolucent shadow results. This shadow may partially obscure the anterior teeth. If the tongue is not kept in contact with the hard palate during the entire exposure, a dark radiolucent shadow obscures the apices of the maxillary anterior teeth (Fig. 4–21).

Solution

In order to prevent lip and tongue positioning errors, the operator should instruct the patient to place their lips on the bite block during the *entire* exposure and to place the tongue on the roof of the mouth. The patient should also be instructed to swallow just before the exposure in order to eliminate the dark radiolucent air space artifact.

Occlusal Plane/Chin Tipped Up

Problem

If the patient's chin is positioned too high (tipped up) and the ala-tragus line is angled upward (instead of 5 degrees downward) (Fig. 4–22), a number of diagnostic problems result. The hard palate and the inferior border of the nasal cavity appear superimposed over the apices of the maxillary teeth, and a loss of information concerning the apical region of the maxillary inci-

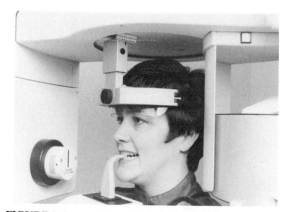

FIGURE 4–19. The patient's teeth must be positioned in the grooves on the bite block.

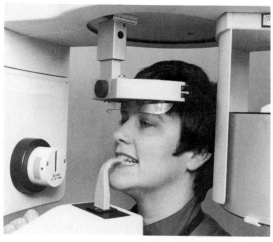

FIGURE 4–22. The patient's head is incorrectly positioned; the chin is tipped up.

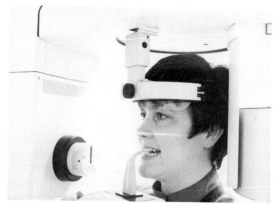

FIGURE 4–20. The patient's Frankfort plane must be positioned so that it is parallel to the floor.

sors results. Because the chin is tipped up, the maxillary incisors are positioned more posteriorly and, as a result, appear blurred and magnified on the panoramic radiograph.

The excessive upward angulation of the chin may also result in the omission of the mandibular condyles from the edges of the film. When a patient's chin is tipped up, a "reverse smile line" or a flat occlusal plane is apparent on the panoramic radiograph (Fig. 4–23).

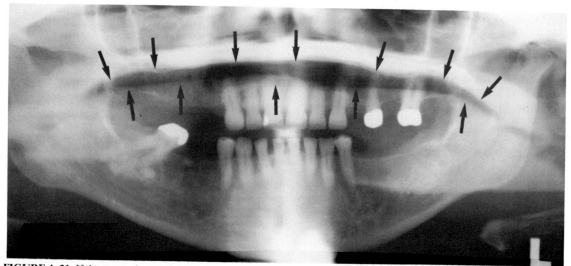

FIGURE 4–21. If the tongue is not placed on the roof of the mouth, a radiolucent shadow will be seen superimposed over the apices of the maxillary teeth.

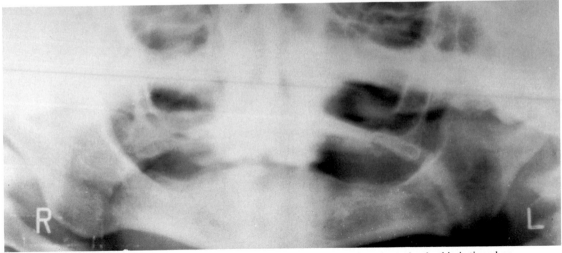

FIGURE 4–23. A "reverse smile line" is seen on a panoramic film when the patient's chin is tipped up.

Solution

The operator must carefully position the patient's head and confirm both the angulations of the ala-tragus line (5 degrees downward) and the Frankfort plane (parallel with the floor) before exposing the film.

Occlusal Plane/Chin Tipped Down

Problem

If the patient's chin is positioned too low (tipped down) and the Frankfort plane is not parallel with the floor (Fig. 4–24), diagnostic problems occur. As a result of the chin position, the mandibular incisors are positioned more posteriorly and appear blurred and exhibit loss of definition in the apical regions. With a downward chin position, the mandibular condyles may either appear to be positioned higher on the film or omitted from the film's upper edge. When a patient's chin is tipped down, the resultant panoramic radiograph exhibits an "exaggerated smile" appearance (Fig. 4–25).

Solution

Once again, the operator must carefully position the patient's head and verify both the angulations of the ala-tragus line and the Frankfort horizontal plane before exposing the film.

Teeth Anterior to the Focal Trough

Problem

Special attention must be taken to align the patient's teeth in the focal trough in order to attain an acceptable panoramic radiograph. The **focal trough** is a three-dimensional horseshoe-shaped zone in which structures can be clearly reproduced. The areas that lie outside of the focal trough appear out of focus. If the patient's anterior teeth are not positioned in the focal trough, the teeth appear blurred and information is lost. The patient's teeth must be properly placed in

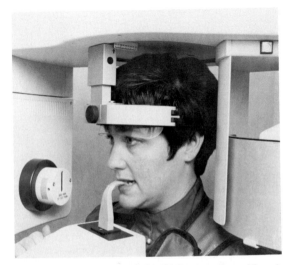

FIGURE 4–24. The patient's head is incorrectly positioned; the chin is tipped down.

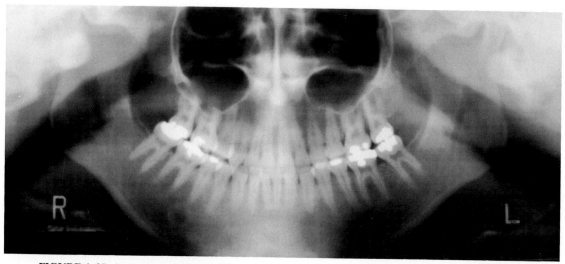

FIGURE 4–25. An "exaggerated smile" is seen on a panoramic film when the patient's chin is tipped down.

the bite groove on the bite block. If the patient's anterior teeth are positioned too far forward on the bite block, that is, anterior to the focal trough (Fig. 4–26), the anterior teeth appear narrowed and blurred. Both the maxillary and mandibular teeth appear "skinny" and out of focus (Fig. 4–27). In addition, the cervical spine is superimposed on the ramus areas and the premolars appear overlapped.

Solution

The operator should position the patient so the anterior teeth are placed in an end-to-end position biting in the bite block groove. The operator should make certain the anterior guide bar is supporting the patient's forehead in order to prevent the patient from moving forward on the bite block and out of the focal trough. Lastly, the operator should remind the patient to remain closed on the bite block during the entire exposure and to hold very still.

Teeth Posterior to the Focal Trough
Problem

As previously stated, if the patient's anterior teeth are not positioned in the focal trough, the teeth appear blurred and information is lost. If the patient's anterior teeth are positioned too far back on the bite block, that is, posterior to the focal trough (Fig. 4–28), the anterior teeth ap-

pear widened and blurred. Both the maxillary and mandibular teeth appear "fat," or magnified, and out of focus (Fig. 4–29). In addition, loss of information concerning the anterior apical regions result. The mandibular condyles may appear partially omitted from the edges of the film resulting in the loss of information concerning the temporomandibular joint areas.

Solution

The operator should position the patient so the anterior teeth are placed in an end-to-end position biting in the bite block groove. The operator should remind the patient to keep the teeth closed on the bite block during the entire exposure and to hold very still.

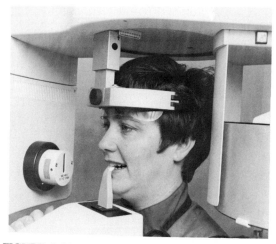

FIGURE 4–26. The patient is incorrectly positioned; the teeth are too far forward on the bite block.

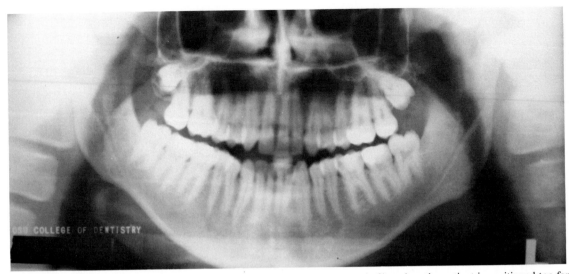

FIGURE 4-27. The anterior teeth appear narrowed and blurred on a panoramic film when the patient is positioned too far forward on the bite block.

Head Tipped, Tilted or Off-Center

Problem

If the patient's head is tipped, tilted or off-center, midsagittal plane positioning errors are seen (Fig. 4–30). If the patient's midsagittal plane is not positioned perpendicular with the floor, the ramus and posterior teeth appear unequally magnified (Fig. 4–31). As a result, a narrow ramus is seen on one side of the panoramic radiograph and a wider ramus is seen on the other side. The side farthest from the film appears magnified, and conversely, the side closest to the film appears smaller.

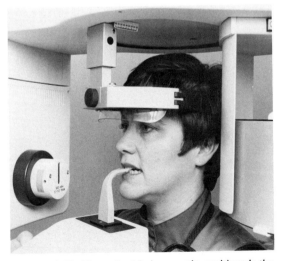

FIGURE 4-28. The patient is incorrectly positioned; the teeth are too far back and not on the bite block.

Solution

The operator must position the patient's head carefully and confirm that the midsagittal plane is perpendicular with the floor. The operator must make certain that the side guide bars are in firm contact with the sides of the patient's head.

Vertebral Column

Problem

The patient's back must be straight and erect. Slouching or slumping results in the increased amount of cervical spine exhibited on the panoramic film (Fig. 4–32). The cervical spine appears as an area of increased radiopacity in the center of the film that may obscure important information.

Solution

The operator should request that the patient stand (or sit) up as tall and as straight as possible. By instructing the patient in this manner, the operator avoids a spinal column positioning error and the resultant nondiagnostic area in the middle of the panoramic radiograph.

THE PANORAMIC FILM AND THE DENTAL PROFESSIONAL

The panoramic radiograph is a valuable diagnostic aid that allows the dental professional to view

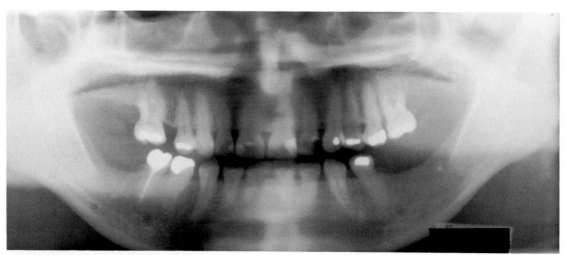

FIGURE 4–29. The anterior teeth appear widened and blurred on a panoramic film when the patient is positioned too far back on the bite block.

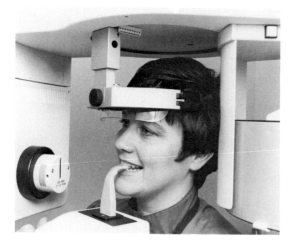

FIGURE 4–30. The patient is incorrectly positioned; the head is tilted off-center.

the entire maxillomandibular region on a single film. The panoramic film is a popular film because of its ease and simplicity of operation and exposure, the reduced radiation exposure to the patient and the anatomic images produced.

In order to produce panoramic radiographs with consistent image quality, operator errors must be minimized. To avoid common errors, the dental professional must be knowledgeable about patient preparation and positioning. In addition, the dental professional must be adequately trained to operate the panoramic radiography equipment. Careful attention to proper patient preparation and positioning assures the diagnostic value of each film and elminates retakes and nondiagnostic films.

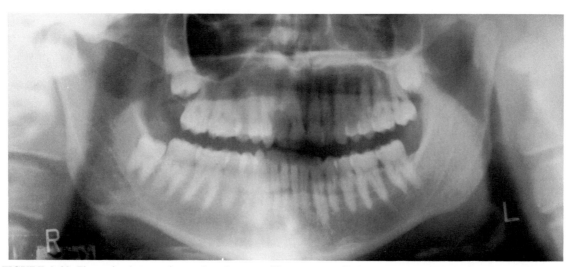

FIGURE 4–31. The patient's posterior teeth and ramus will appear magnified on a panoramic film when the head is tilted off-center.

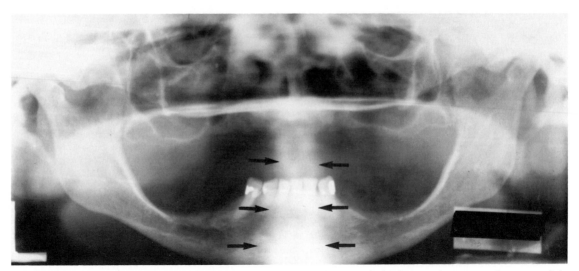

FIGURE 4–32. If the patient is not standing erect, superimposition of the cervical spine may be seen on the center of the panoramic film.

SUMMARY

The panoramic radiograph is an ideal way for the dental professional to view a large area of the maxilla and mandible on a single film. Recognition of normal anatomic landmarks is necessary for interpretation of panoramic radiographs. A knowledge of normal anatomy viewed on panoramic radiographs is essential before the dental professional can begin to recognize what is abnormal.

Chapter 4 has reviewed the normal anatomic landmarks of the maxilla and mandible, air space images, soft tissue images and artifacts seen on panoramic radiographs as well as common panoramic positioning errors.

Bibliography

Brand RW and Isselhard DE: Osteology of the skull. *In* Anatomy of Orofacial Structures, 4th ed., pp 117–33. St. Louis: CV Mosby, 1990.

Dental Auxiliary Education Project: Normal Radiographic Landmarks. New York: Teachers College Press, 1982.

Langland OE, et al.: Panoramic Radiology, 2d ed., pp 224–71. Philadelphia: Lea and Febiger, 1989.

QUIZ QUESTIONS

"What Can This Be?"

1. Identify the normal anatomical features in Figure 4–33 labeled 1 to 15.

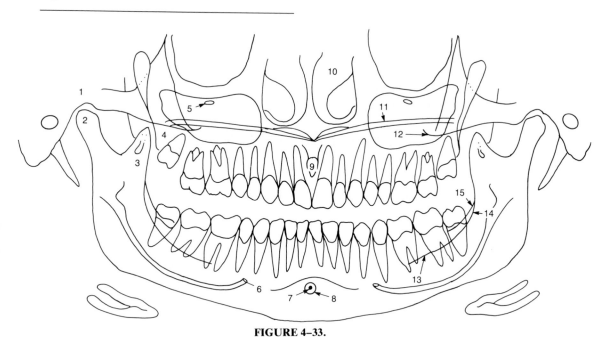

FIGURE 4–33.

2. Identify the normal anatomical feature in Figure 4–34 labeled 1 to 16.

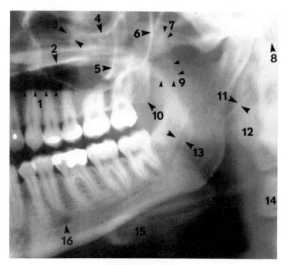

FIGURE 4–34.

Matching

Match the following error with the potential cause.

___ **3.** Ghost image   A. Anterior teeth appear "fat"

___ **4.** Teeth anterior to focal trough   B. Reverse smile line

___ **5.** Lips open during exposure   C. Radiopaque streak blurred across film

___ **6.** Chin tipped down   D. Radiolucency obscuring anterior teeth

___ **7.** Patient slumped   E. Anterior teeth appear "skinny"

___ **8.** Teeth posterior to focal trough   F. Exaggerated smile

___ **9.** Improper lead apron placement   G. Radiopaque cone-shaped artifact

___ **10.** Chin tipped up   H. Increased radiopacity in center of film

CHAPTER FIVE

Identification of Restorations, Dental Materials and Foreign Objects

Objectives   After completion of this chapter, the student will be able to:

▶ Discuss the importance of interpreting radiographs while the patient is present.

▶ Identify and describe the radiographic appearance of the following restorations: amalgam, gold, stainless steel and chrome, post and core, porcelain, porcelain-fused-to-metal, composite and acrylic.

▶ Identify and describe the radiographic appearance of the following dental materials and devices: base materials, metallic pins, gutta percha, silver points, removable partial dentures, complete dentures, orthodontic bands, brackets and wires, fixed retainers, implants, suture wires, splints and stabilizing arches and wires.

▶ Identify and describe the radiographic appearance of the following miscellaneous objects: jewelry, eyeglasses and patient napkin chains.

▶ Define the buccal object rule.

▶ Identify illustrations concerning the buccal object rule.

Key Words   **Buccal object rule**   **Nonmetallic restoration**
                     Diatoric   **Radiolucent**
                     Ghost image   **Radiopaque**
                     Metallic restoration

Dental radiographs are an important diagnostic tool that enables the practitioner to view dental restorations and materials. Radiographs are also useful in identifying and locating foreign objects. Some restorations, materials and foreign objects are easily identified on dental radiographs; others are not. The radiographic appearance of restorations, materials and foreign objects varies depending on the material's thickness, density and atomic number. Some restorations, materials and foreign objects may be identified by the degree of radiopacity present, outline, contour or size; others require additional clinical information.

All dental radiographs should be interpreted by the dental professional while the patient is present. If questions arise as to what is seen on a radiograph concerning dental restorations, materials or foreign objects, examination of the patient can be used to obtain additional information or to verify what is seen radiographically. If radiographs are interpreted without the patient present, some important clinical information is not available.

The purpose of this chapter is to review common dental restorations, materials and foreign objects that may be seen on dental radiographs and to explore the use of the buccal object rule as a localization technique.

IDENTIFICATION OF RESTORATIONS

A variety of common restorative materials, including amalgam, gold, stainless steel, porcelain, composite and acrylic can be identified on dental radiographs.

Metallic restorations (e.g., amalgam and gold) absorb x-rays, and as a result, very little (if any) radiation comes in contact with the film. Consequently, that area of the film remains unexposed and the metallic restorations appear completely radiopaque on a dental radiograph. To illustrate the fact that a completely radiopaque area on a processed film represents an unexposed portion of the film, place a radiograph with a metallic restoration on a printed page. The underlying print can be easily read through the radiopaque area on the film (Fig. 5–1).

Nonmetallic restorations (e.g., porcelain, composite and acrylic) may vary in radiographic appearance from radiolucent to slightly radiopaque depending on the density of the material. Of the nonmetallic restorations, porcelain is the most dense and least radiolucent, and acrylic is the least dense and most radiolucent.

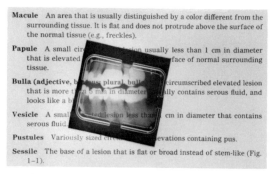

Macule   An area that is usually distinguished by a color different from the surrounding tissue. It is flat and does not protrude above the surface of the normal tissue (e.g., freckles).

Papule   A small cir... ...ion usually less than 1 cm in diameter that is elevated ...face of normal surrounding tissue.

Bulla (adjective, b... ...us plural, bull... ...circumscribed elevated lesion that is more t... ...an 5 mm in diameter ...lly contains serous fluid, and looks like a b...

Vesicle   A smal... ...ed lesion less than ...cm in diameter that contains serous fluid.

Pustules   Variously sized cir... ...evations containing pus.

Sessile   The base of a lesion that is flat or broad instead of stem-like (Fig. 1–1).

FIGURE 5–1. When a radiograph with a metallic restoration is placed on a printed page, the print can be easily seen.

Amalgam Restorations

Amalgam is the most common restorative material used in dentistry. Amalgam absorbs the x-ray beam and prevents x-rays from reaching the film; consequently, amalgam appears completely radiopaque on a dental radiograph. Amalgam may be seen in a variety of shapes, sizes and locations on a dental radiograph.

One-Surface Amalgam Restorations

One-surface amalgam restorations (pit amalgams) appear as distinct, small round or ovoid radiopacities (Figs. 5–2 and 5–3). One-surface amalgams may be seen on the buccal, lingual or occlusal surfaces of the teeth. Larger two-surface and multi-surface amalgam restorations also appear radiopaque and are characterized by their irregular outlines or borders (Figs. 5–4 and 5–5). Multi-surface amalgam restorations may involve any tooth surface.

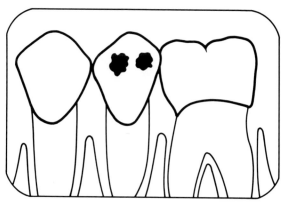

FIGURE 5–2. Pit amalgam.

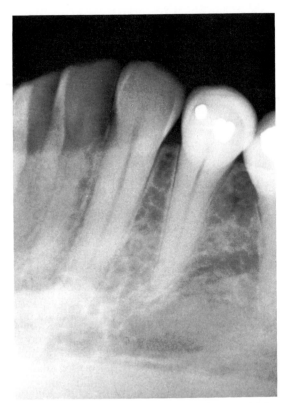

FIGURE 5–3. Two tiny pit amalgams seen in a mandibular premolar.

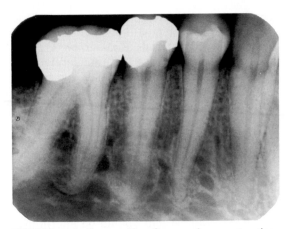

FIGURE 5–5. Two multi-surface amalgam restorations. (Note the irregular outlines.)

Amalgam Overhangs

Amalgam overhangs can be described as extensions of amalgam seen beyond the crown portion of a tooth located in the interproximal region. An amalgam overhang results from improper band placement around a tooth prior to the condensing of the amalgam restoration. Amalgam overhangs can be easily visualized on a dental radiograph and appear radiopaque (Figs. 5–6 and 5–7). An amalgam overhang dis-

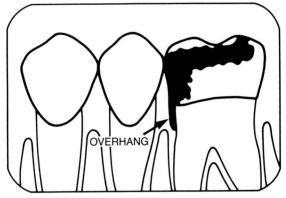

FIGURE 5–6. An amalgam overhang.

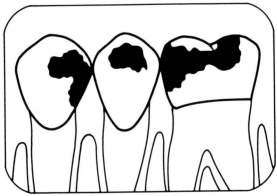

FIGURE 5–4. A multi-surface amalgam.

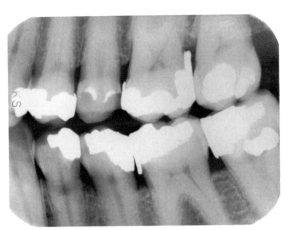

FIGURE 5–7. Amalgam overhangs seen on the maxillary first molar and mandibular first and second molars.

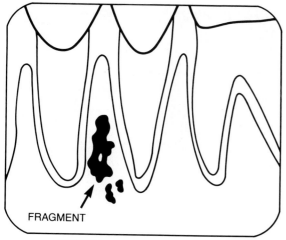

FIGURE 5–8. Amalgam fragments.

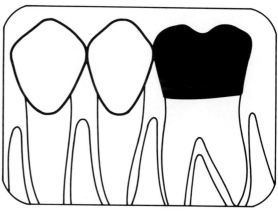

FIGURE 5–10. A gold crown.

rupts the natural cleansing contours of the tooth, traps food and plaque and contributes to bone loss. In order to prevent destruction of interproximal bone, amalgam overhangs must be removed.

Amalgam Fragments

Fragments of amalgam may be inadvertently embedded in adjacent soft tissue during the restoration of a tooth. Amalgam fragments or scraps vary in size and shape and appear as dense radiopacities with irregular borders on a dental radiograph (Figs. 5–8 and 5–9). Amalgam fragments may be seen anywhere there is soft tissue.

Gold Restorations

It is not always possible to differentiate one metallic restoration from another on a dental radio-

graph; however, an educated guess is often possible if the shape and size of the restoration is considered. Both gold and amalgam appear equally radiopaque on a dental radiograph. A large radiopaque restoration with smooth borders is most probably gold. Gold restorations appear completely radiopaque and, unlike amalgam restorations, exhibit a smooth marginal outline (Figs. 5–10 and 5–11). If dental radiographs are interpreted with the patient present, examination of the patient can be used to obtain additional information concerning gold versus amalgam or to verify what is seen radiographically.

Gold Crowns and Bridges

Gold crowns and bridges appear as large radiopaque restorations with smooth contours and regular borders (Fig. 5–12). Similarly, gold inlays and onlays exhibit marginal outlines that

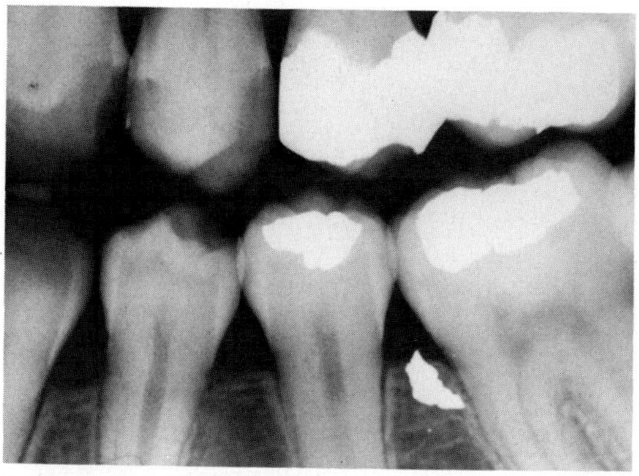

FIGURE 5–9. Amalgam fragment seen between the mandibular second premolar and the first molar.

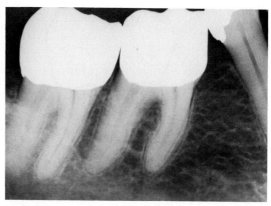

FIGURE 5–11. Two gold crowns on the mandibular molars. (Note the smooth outline and contour.)

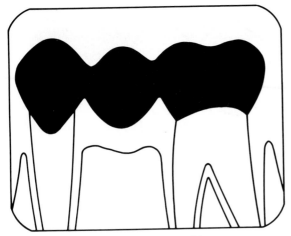

FIGURE 5–12. A gold bridge.

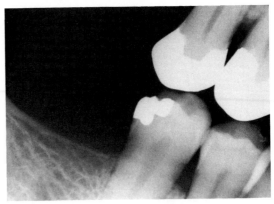

FIGURE 5–14. Gold onlays on the maxillary premolars. (Note the distinct outline and contours.)

appear smooth and regular (Figs. 5–13 and 5–14).

Gold Foil Restorations

Gold foil restorations (one-surface) appear as small round radiopacities on a dental radiograph and are indistinguishable from the one-surface amalgam restorations. A two-surface gold foil restoration may appear similar to the gold inlay, with smooth, regular marginal outlines or exhibit slightly irregular margins and resemble the two-surface amalgam.

Stainless Steel and Chrome Crowns

Stainless steel and chrome crowns are prefabricated restorations that are usually used as interim or temporary restorations. These crowns

are thin and do not absorb dental x-rays to the extent that amalgam, gold and other cast metals do. As a result, both stainless steel and chrome crowns appear radiopaque, but not as densely radiopaque as amalgam or gold.

Stainless steel and chrome crowns appear radiopaque on a dental radiograph. These crowns are prefabricated, and their outlines and margins appear very smooth and regular. Often these crowns are not contoured properly to the cervical portion of the tooth and, as a result, do not appear to fit the tooth well (Fig. 5–15). Because stainless steel and chrome crowns are thin, some areas may appear "see-through" (Fig. 5–16).

Post and Core Restorations

Post and core restorations can be seen in endodontically treated teeth. The post and core restoration is cast metal and appears as radiodense as amalgam or gold. Post and core restorations

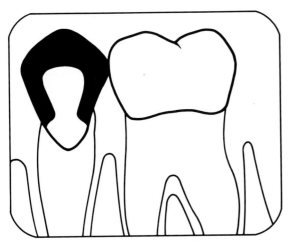

FIGURE 5–13. A gold onlay.

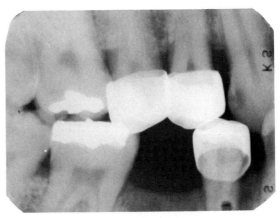

FIGURE 5–15. Three stainless steel crowns.

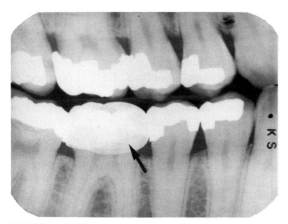

FIGURE 5–16. A stainless steel crown on the mandibular first molar. (Note the area that appears "see-through.")

appear radiopaque on a dental radiograph. The core portion of the restoration resembles the prepped portion of a tooth crown, and the post portion extends into the pulp canal (Fig. 5–17).

Porcelain Restorations

A porcelain restoration appears radiopaque on a dental radiograph. Unlike metallic restorations, which appear totally radiopaque, porcelain res-

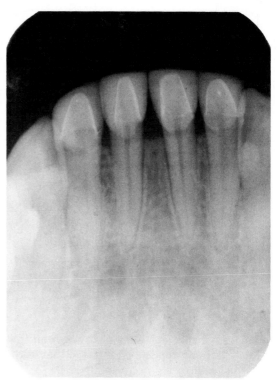

FIGURE 5–18. Porcelain crowns seen on the mandibular anterior teeth. (Note the outline of the tooth preparation covered with radiopaque cement.)

torations are slightly radiopaque and resemble the radiodensity of dentin.

All-Porcelain Crowns

All-porcelain crowns appear slightly radiopaque on a dental radiograph (Fig. 5–18). A thin radiopaque line outlining the prepared tooth may be evident through the slightly radiopaque porcelain crown (Fig. 5–19). This thin line repre-

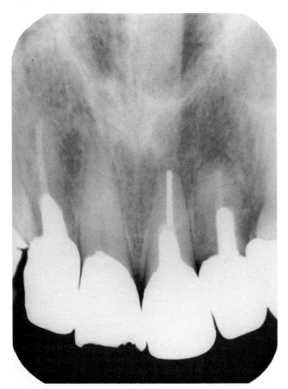

FIGURE 5–17. Post and core restorations seen on the maxillary anterior teeth.

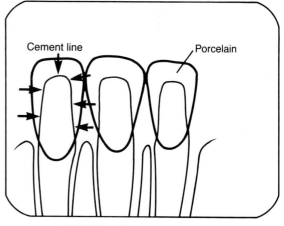

FIGURE 5–19. A porcelain crown.

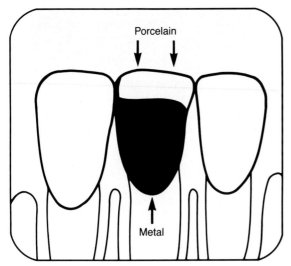

FIGURE 5–20. A porcelain-fused-to-metal crown.

sents cement. The radiodensity of an all-porcelain bridge appears identical to that of the all-porcelain crown.

Porcelain-Fused-to-Metal Crown

A porcelain-fused-to-metal crown has two radiographic components. The metal component appears completely radiopaque and the porcelain component appears slightly radiopaque (Figs. 5–20 and 5–21). The radiodensities of a porcelain-fused-to-metal bridge appear identical to that seen in the porcelain-fused-to-metal crown (Fig. 5–22).

Composite Restorations

A composite restoration may vary in radiographic appearance from radiolucent to slightly radiopaque, depending on the composition of the composite material (Figs. 5–23 and 5–24). Some manufacturers of composite materials add radiopaque particles to their products in order to help the viewer differentiate a composite restoration from dental caries (which appear radiolucent) on a dental radiograph.

Should the question arise concerning a composite restoration versus dental caries, a careful visual and digital examination of the tooth in question enables the clinician to distinguish between the two.

Acrylic Restorations

Acrylic resin restorations are often used as an interim or temporary crown or filling. Of all the nonmetallic restorations, acrylic is the least dense and appears radiolucent or barely visible on a dental radiograph.

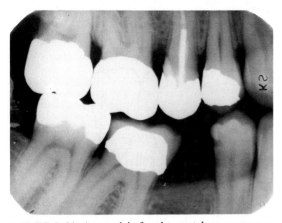

FIGURE 5–21. A porcelain-fused-to-metal crown seen on the mandibular first molar.

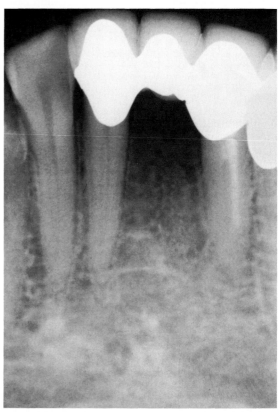

FIGURE 5–22. A porcelain-fused-to-metal bridge seen in the mandibular anterior region.

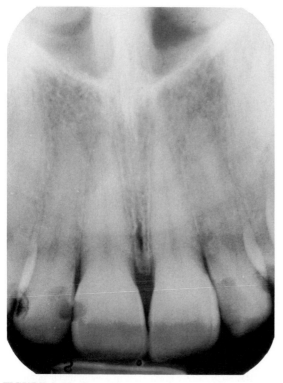

FIGURE 5-23. Composite restorations seen on maxillary anterior teeth.

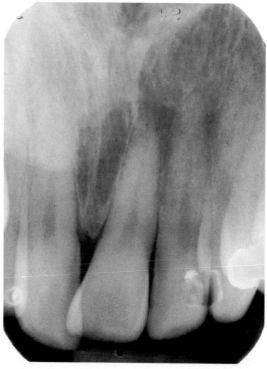

FIGURE 5-24. Composite restorations seen on maxillary anterior teeth. (Note the slight radiopaque appearance.)

IDENTIFICATION OF MATERIALS USED IN DENTISTRY

A number of materials are used in dentistry for a variety of reasons, each specific to the specialty that requires them. Practitioners in restorative dentistry, endodontics, prosthodontics, orthodontics and oral surgery all use materials that can be identified on dental radiographs.

Materials Used in Restorative Dentistry

Base Materials

Base materials, which include zinc phosphate cement and zinc oxide–eugenol paste, are used as cavity liners to protect the pulp of the tooth. Base materials are placed on the floor of a cavity preparation. A restorative material, such as amalgam, is then placed over the base material. A base material appears radiopaque. If compared with amalgam, the base material appears less radiodense (Fig. 5–25).

Metallic Pins

Metallic pins, used to enhance the retention of amalgam or composite, appear as cylindrical or screw-shaped radiopacities on a dental radiograph (Fig. 5–26).

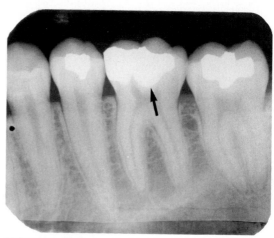

FIGURE 5-25. Base material seen under an amalgam restoration on a mandibular first molar.

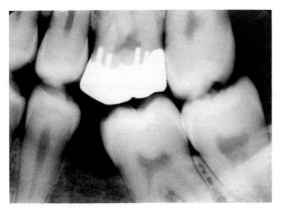

FIGURE 5–26. Maxillary molar seen with four retention pins.

Materials Used in Endodontics

Gutta Percha

Gutta percha is a clay-like material used in endodontic therapy to fill the pulp canals. Gutta percha appears radiopaque, similar in density to that of base materials (Fig. 5–27). When compared with metallic restorations, gutta percha appears less radiodense.

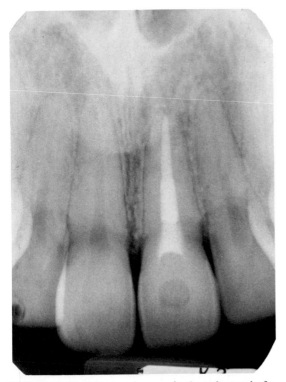

FIGURE 5–27. Gutta percha seen in the pulp canal of a maxillary central incisor.

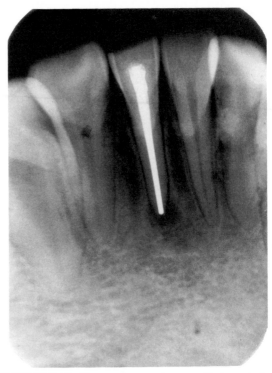

FIGURE 5–28. Silver point seen in a mandibular anterior tooth.

Silver Points

Silver points are also used in endodontic therapy to fill pulp canals. Silver points appear very radiopaque, similar to other metallic materials. Silver points appear more radiodense than gutta percha (Fig. 5–28).

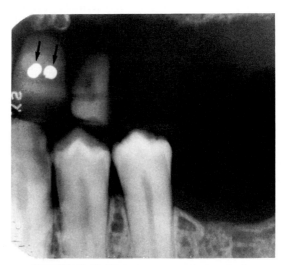

FIGURE 5–29. Diatorics seen on denture teeth.

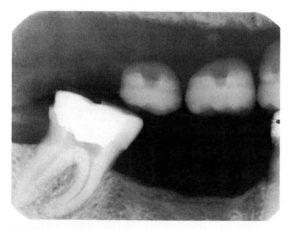

FIGURE 5–30. Maxillary denture teeth appear to be "floating" in this bite-wing radiograph.

Materials Used in Prosthodontics

Complete and removable partial dentures are common and may be occasionally observed on dental radiographs. The radiographic appearance of complete and removable partial dentures varies depending on the base materials and type of denture teeth used.

Patients should be instructed to remove all complete and partial dentures before dental radiographs are taken. If not removed, complete and partial dentures may obscure important information concerning adjacent teeth and underlying bone.

Complete Dentures

A complete denture consists of two component parts: a base material and denture teeth. The typical denture base material is composed of acrylic and appears as a very faint radiopacity on a dental radiograph or, in some instances, may not be seen at all. Denture teeth may be porcelain or acrylic and vary in their radiographic appearance. Porcelain denture teeth appear radiopaque and resemble the radiodensity of dentin. Anterior porcelain denture teeth include one or two metal retention pins, or **diatorics.** On a dental radiograph, the diatorics appear as tiny dense radiopacities superimposed over the radiopaque porcelain denture teeth (Fig. 5–29). Posterior porcelain denture teeth also appear radiopaque but do not contain diatorics. Acrylic (plastic) denture teeth lack density and appear faintly radiopaque or radiolucent on a dental radiograph.

A complete denture that is not removed before the exposure of a dental radiograph gives the illusion of rootless, or floating, teeth (Fig. 5–30).

Removable Partial Dentures

A removable partial denture can be constructed from a variety of base materials, including cast metal, a combination of cast metal and acrylic, or all acrylic. The removable partial denture constructed of cast metal appears densely radiopaque on a radiograph. The size and shape of the radiopacity depends on the design of the

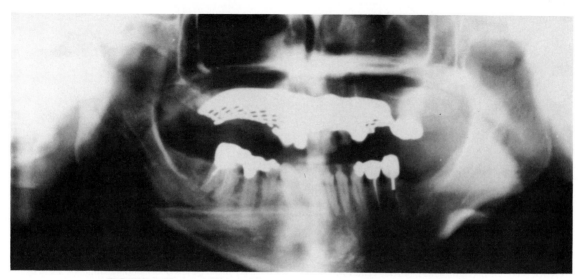

FIGURE 5–31. A maxillary removable partial denture seen on a panoramic film.

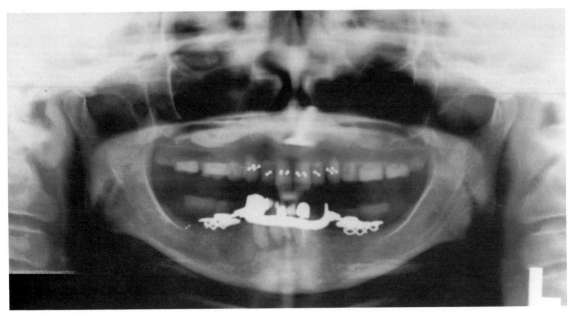

FIGURE 5–32. The teeth on the mandibular partial denture appear slightly radiopaque on this radiograph.

metal framework of the partial denture (Fig. 5–31). A removable partial denture constructed of a metal base with acrylic saddles appears densely radiopaque where metal is present and slightly radiopaque in the areas of acrylic. A removable partial denture base constructed totally of acrylic is usually seen with wrought metal clasps. The acrylic base appears slightly radiopaque or radiolucent on a dental radiograph. The metal clasps appear radiopaque and are seen resting on abutment teeth.

Teeth in a removable partial denture may be composed of either acrylic or porcelain. Porcelain teeth appear radiopaque and resemble the radiodensity of dentin. Acrylic teeth appear faintly radiopaque or radiolucent (Fig. 5–32).

Materials Used in Orthodontics

Orthodontic bands, brackets and wires may be observed on dental radiographs. These ortho-

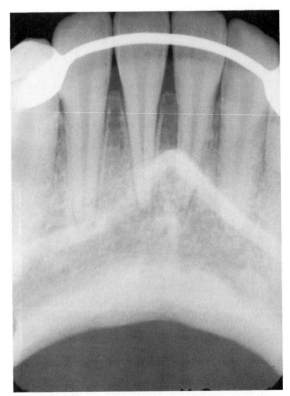

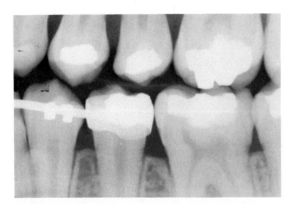

FIGURE 5–33. Orthodontic bands, brackets and wires seen on mandibular teeth.

FIGURE 5–34. A fixed orthodontic retainer seen in the mandibular anterior region.

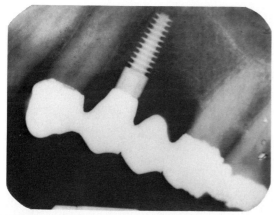

FIGURE 5–35. An implant serves as support for a maxillary bridge.

dontic materials have a characteristic radiopaque appearance (Fig. 5–33). Fixed orthodontic retainers may also be observed on dental radiographs and have an equally characteristic appearance (Fig. 5–34).

Materials Used in Oral Surgery

Implants are being used in oral surgery with increased frequency. A number of endosteal implants exist, and the radiographic appearance varies based on the shape and design of the implant used. The endosteal implant is made out of a metallic material and appears radiopaque on a dental radiograph (Fig. 5–35).

Suture wires, metallic splints and plates and stabilizing arches are used in oral surgery to stabilize fractures of the maxilla and mandible. Suture wires appear as thin radiopaque lines (Fig. 5–36). Metallic splints, plates and stabilizing arches also appear radiopaque; their shape and size vary (Figs. 5–37 and 5–38).

IDENTIFICATION OF MISCELLANEOUS OBJECTS

A number of miscellaneous objects, such as jewelry, eyeglasses and patient napkin chains can be viewed on dental radiographs. Such miscellaneous objects may obscure important diagnostic information. Some miscellaneous objects may be seen on intraoral radiographs, while others may be noted on extraoral films.

In order to avoid nondiagnostic films, patients should be instructed to remove earrings, necklaces, nose jewelry, eyeglasses and patient napkin chains before the exposure of extraoral films. With intraoral films, patients should be instructed to remove eyeglasses and nose jewelry, if necessary.

Jewelry

Earrings most often appear on extraoral films. Metal earrings appear as dense radiopacities on a dental radiograph; the size and shape of the radiopacity corresponds to the size and shape of the earring (Figs. 5–39 and 5–40). Plastic earrings with metallic posts and backings or metal clips can also be seen on dental radiographs; the

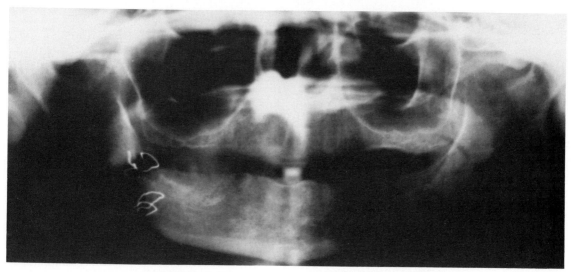

FIGURE 5–36. Two suture wires seen in the posterior mandible.

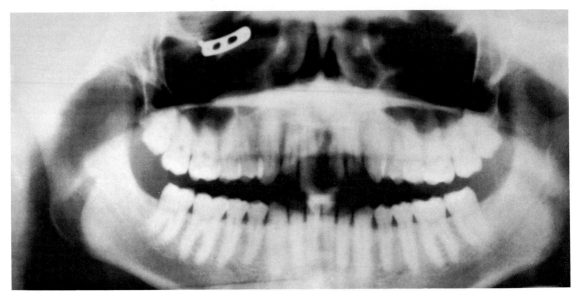

FIGURE 5–37. A small metal plate with screws seen in the region of the orbit.

metallic portions appear as dense radiopacities. A radiodense object, such as a metal earring, causes an artifact on panoramic films known as a **ghost image** (see Chapter 4). Ghost images can obscure important information about the teeth and bones and render the film nondiagnostic (Fig. 5–41).

Necklaces may also appear on extraoral films as a radiopacity that corresponds in shape and size to the jewelry (Fig. 5–42). Nose jewelry (small studs or hoop earrings worn on the nose) may also be seen on extraoral radiographs or intraoral films (e.g., maxillary anterior periapicals). This type of jewelry appears as a radiopacity on a dental film and corresponds in size and shape to the object it represents (Fig. 5–43).

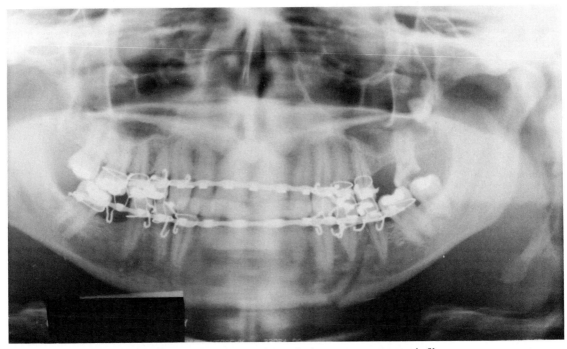

FIGURE 5–38. Stabilizing arches and wires seen on a panoramic film.

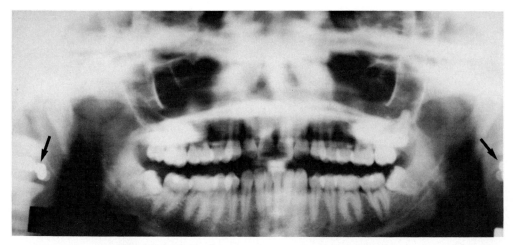

FIGURE 5–39. Small post earrings seen on a panoramic film.

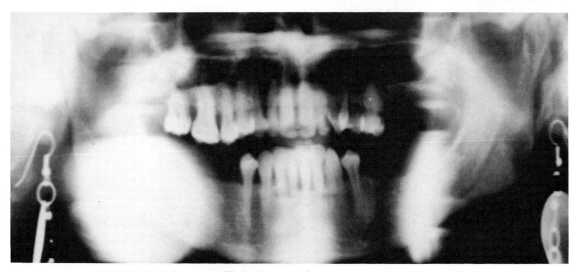

FIGURE 5–40. Large metallic earrings and ghost images seen on a panoramic film.

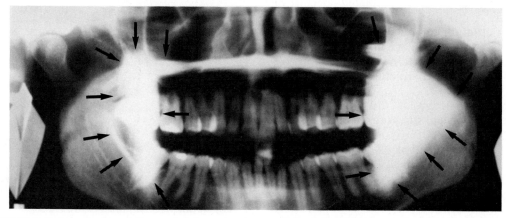

FIGURE 5–41. Note the loss of diagnostic information that results from the ghost images of the large metallic earrings.

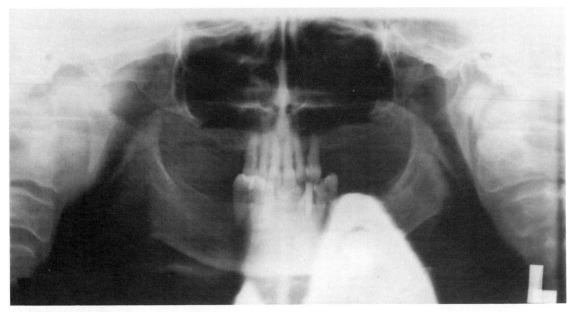

FIGURE 5–42. A metallic necklace may appear as a radiopaque loop in the region of the mandible.

Miscellaneous

Eyeglasses may also be seen on extraoral and intraoral films. Most eyeglasses have some metal components in the frames. The metal portion of the frames appears as a radiopacity on a dental film (Fig. 5–44).

The patient napkin chain, similar to a necklace, may be seen on an extraoral radiograph. A radiopacity resembling the napkin chain is seen on the film (Fig. 5–45).

THE BUCCAL OBJECT RULE

It is sometimes necessary to determine if structures or foreign objects are situated buccally or lingually. A quick and easy method for determining this information is the **buccal object rule,** which is a localization technique that allows the practitioner to determine the position of superimposed dental structures or foreign objects.

In order to determine the location of the superimposed dental structures in question, *two* radiographs need to be exposed utilizing different horizontal angulations. The different horizontal angulations (or change in the direction of the x-ray beam) correspond with a change in the position of the object on the radiograph.

One intraoral radiograph is exposed using proper technique and angulation; a second radiograph is then exposed after the tubehead and corresponding direction of the x-ray beam has been changed. If the dental structure or object seen on the second radiograph appears to have moved in the *same direction as the shift of the*

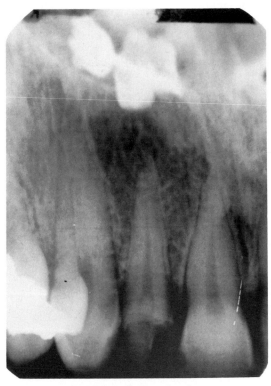

FIGURE 5–43. Nose jewelry.

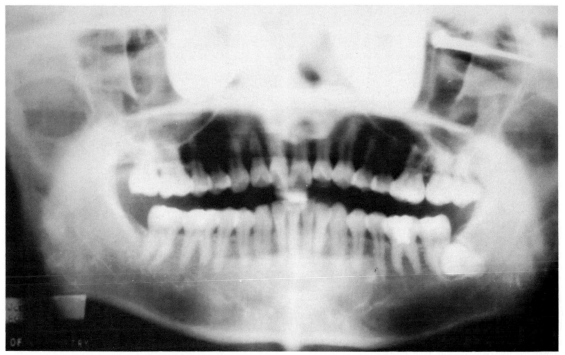

FIGURE 5–44. Eyeglasses seen on a panoramic film.

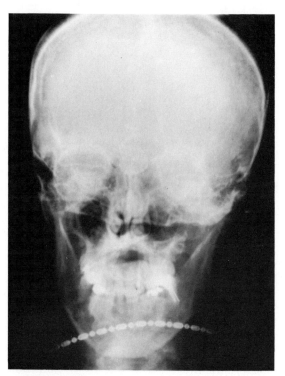

FIGURE 5–45. Napkin chain seen on a posterior-anterior skull film.

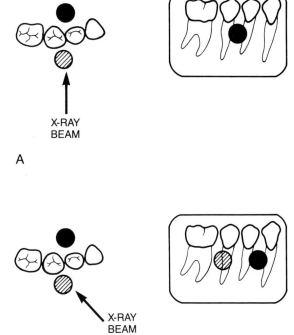

A

B

FIGURE 5–46. Buccal and lingual objects shift positions when the direction of the x-ray beam is changed. *A*, Buccal (*crosshatched circle*) and lingual (*black circle*) are superimposed in the original radiograph. *B*, If the tubehead is shifted in a mesial direction, the buccal object moves distally and the lingual object moves mesially. (Same direction = lingual; opposite direction = buccal.)

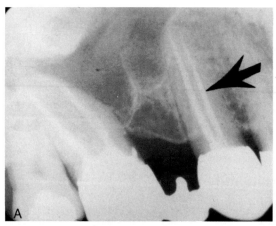
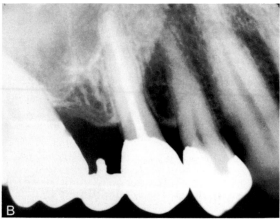

FIGURE 5–47. *A*, Notice the two canals filled with gutta percha in the maxillary second premolar (*arrow*). *B*, The tubehead was shifted in a mesial direction, and the gutta percha moved in a distal direction. The gutta percha is buccal. (Radiographs courtesy of Dr. Robert Jaynes, Assistant Professor, Section of Diagnostic Services, The Ohio State University College of Dentistry.)

tube, then the structure or object in question is located on the *lingual* aspect. For example, if the tubehead is shifted mesially and the object in question appears to move mesially on the radiograph, then the object lies to the lingual (Figs. 5–46 and 5–47).

Conversely, if the dental structure or object seen on the second radiograph appears to move in the *opposite direction as the shift of the tube,* then the structure or object in question is located on the *buccal* aspect. For example, if shifting the tubehead distally produces an object that has moved mesially, then the structure or object lies to the buccal (Figs. 5–48 and 5–49).

A mnemonic that can be used to remember the buccal object rule is SLOB, which stands for *s*ame *l*ingual, *o*pposite *b*uccal. In other words, when the two radiographs are compared, the object that lies to the lingual appears to have moved in the same direction as the tube shift, and the object that lies to the buccal appears to have moved in the opposite direction from the tube shift.

SUMMARY

Several types of dental restorations, materials and foreign objects can be seen and evaluated on extraoral and intraoral radiographs. The radiographic appearance of restorations, materials and foreign objects varies depending on the material composition, density and thickness. The radiographic appearance of restorations and materials can range from completely radiopaque (white) to totally radiolucent (black). Some restorations and objects are easily identified on

dental radiographs, while others may require additional clinical information. Radiographs play an important role in the evaluation of dental restorations, materials and objects. In addition,

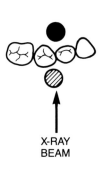
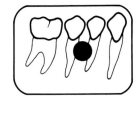

A

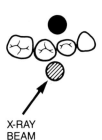
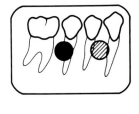

B

FIGURE 5–48. Buccal and lingual objects shift positions when the direction of the x-ray beam is changed. *A*, Buccal (*crosshatched circle*) and lingual (*black circle*) objects are superimposed in the original radiograph. *B*, If the tubehead is shifted in a distal direction, the buccal object moves mesially and the lingual object moves distally. (Same direction = lingual; opposite direction = buccal.)

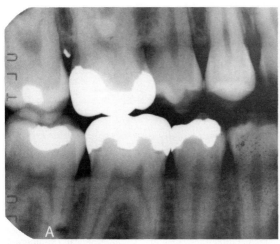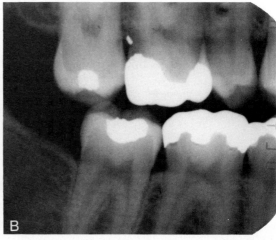

FIGURE 5–49. *A,* Notice the amalgam fragment between the maxillary first and second molars. *B,* The tubehead was shifted in a distal direction, and the amalgam fragment moved in a mesial direction. The amalgam fragment is buccal. (Radiographs courtesy of Dr. Robert Jaynes, Assistant Professor, Section of Diagnostic Services, The Ohio State University College of Dentistry.)

radiographs can be used to localize foreign objects, lesions or teeth viewed on dental films. The buccal object rule, a rule for the orientation of structures portrayed in two or more radiographs exposed at different angles, can be used as a localization technique.

It is important that the dental professional interpret dental radiographs with the patient present. Without the patient present, important clinical information is not available. With the patient present, if there is any question concerning what is seen on a radiograph, a clinical examination can provide additional information or verify what is seen on the dental film.

Bibliography

DeLyre WR and Johnson ON: Preliminary interpretation of the radiographs. *In* Essentials of Dental Radiography for Dental Assistants and Hygienists, 4th ed., pp 179–81, 201–2. Norwalk, CT: Appleton and Lange, 1990.

Frommer HH: Film mounting and normal radiographic anatomy. *In* Radiology for Dental Auxiliaries, 4th ed., pp 238–41. St. Louis: CV Mosby, 1987.

Goaz PW and White SC: Normal radiographic anatomy. *In* Oral Radiology Principles and Interpretation, 2d ed., pp 195–99. St. Louis: CV Mosby, 1987.

Langlais RP and Kasle MJ: Localization techniques. *In* Exercises in Oral Radiographic Interpretation, 3rd ed., pp 147–50. Philadelphia: WB Saunders, 1992.

Langlais RP and Kasle MJ: Identification of materials and foreign objects. *In* Exercises in Oral Radiographic Interpretation, 3rd ed., pp 57–69. Philadelphia: WB Saunders, 1992.

Manson-Hing LR: Intraoral radiographic anatomy and film mounting. *In* Fundamentals of Dental Radiography, 3d ed., p 102. Philadelphia: Lea and Febiger, 1990.

Manson-Hing LR: Fast exposure and localization technics. *In* Fundamentals of Dental Radiography, 3d ed., pp 136–39. Philadelphia: Lea and Febiger, 1990.

Miles DA, et al.: Accessory radiographic techniques and patient management. *In* Radiographic Imaging for Dental Auxiliaries. Philadelphia: WB Saunders, 1989.

QUIZ QUESTIONS

"What Can This Be?"

1. Identify the restoration indicated (Fig. 5–50).

_____

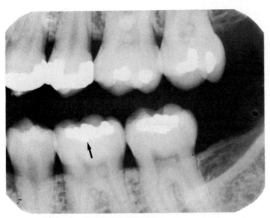

FIGURE 5–50.

3. Identify the restoration indicated (Fig. 5–52).

_____

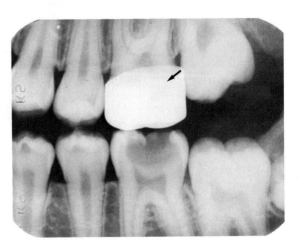

FIGURE 5–52.

2. Identify the restoration indicated (Fig. 5–51).

_____

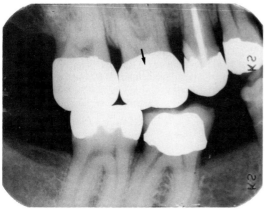

FIGURE 5–51.

4. Identify the dental material indicated (Fig. 5–53).

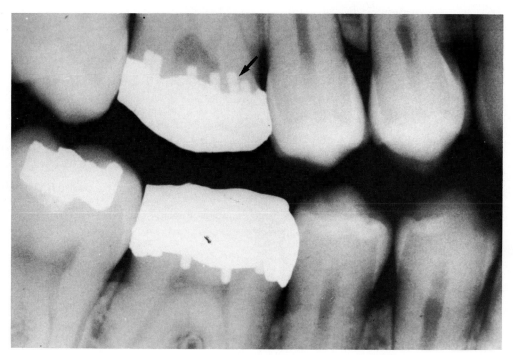

FIGURE 5–53.

5. Identify the dental material indicated (Fig. 5–54).

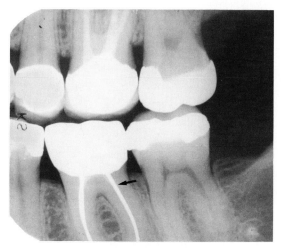

FIGURE 5–54.

6. Identify the object indicated (Fig. 5–55).

_____

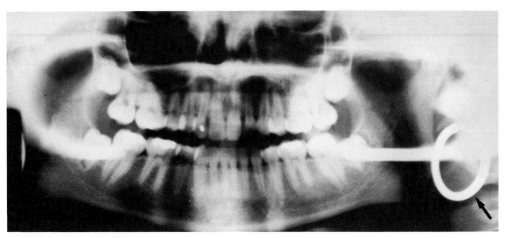

FIGURE 5–55.

7. Identify the object indicated (Fig. 5–56).

_____

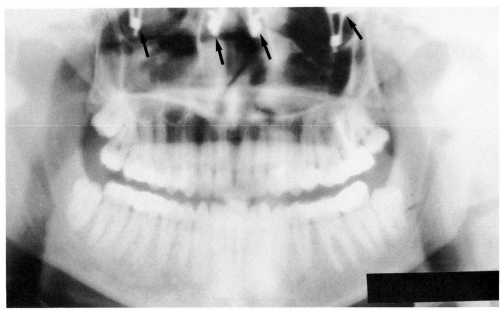

FIGURE 5–56.

8. Why do the teeth in this radiograph appear
to be floating (Fig. 5–57)?

_____

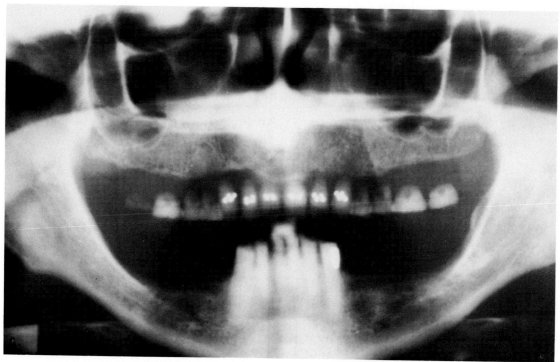

FIGURE 5–57.

9. Using the buccal object rule (Fig. 5–58), is
the pit amalgam buccal or lingual?

_____

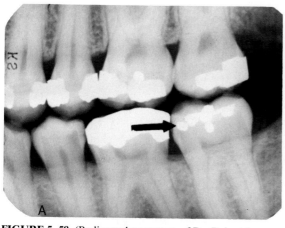 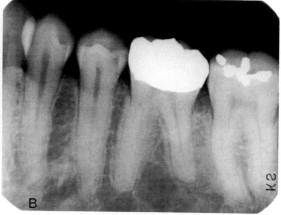

FIGURE 5–58. (Radiographs courtesy of Dr. Robert Jaynes, Assistant Professor, Section of Diagnostic Services, The Ohio State University College of Dentistry.)

10. Using the buccal object rule (Fig. 5–59), is the maxillary canine located buccal or lingual to the adjacent teeth?

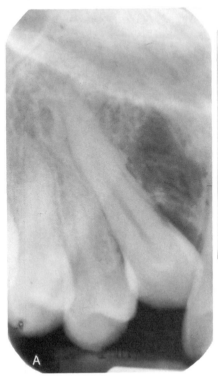

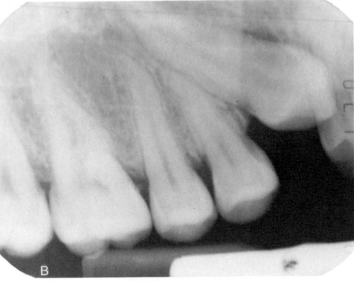

FIGURE 5–59. (Radiographs courtesy of Dr. Robert Jaynes, Assistant Professor, Section of Diagnostic Services, The Ohio State University College of Dentistry.)

Multiple Choice

11. Rank the following restorative materials from most radiopaque (1) to least radiopaque or radiolucent (4).

_____ Gutta percha
_____ Acrylic restorations
_____ Amalgam
_____ Stainless steel crown

12. Which of the following appear *equally* radiopaque on a dental radiograph?
  a. Gold crowns and amalgam
  b. Gold crowns and porcelain crowns
  c. Gutta percha and silver points
  d. Gold crowns and stainless steel crowns

13. Which of the following is *most* radiopaque?
  a. Amalgam
  b. Porcelain
  c. Composite
  d. Acrylic

14. Which of the following is *least* radiopaque?
  a. Amalgam
  b. Porcelain
  c. Stainless steel
  d. Acrylic

15. Which of the following describes how gold can be distinguished from amalgam on a dental radiograph?
  a. Gold appears more radiopaque than amalgam
  b. Gold appears more radiolucent than amalgam
  c. Gold margins are smooth and regular
  d. Amalgam margins are smooth and regular

Short Answer

16. Describe the difference between a gold crown and a stainless steel crown as viewed on a dental radiograph.

17. Describe the difference between gutta percha and silver points as viewed on a dental radiograph.

18. Discuss the importance of interpreting dental radiographs with the patient present.

19. Define the buccal object rule.

CHAPTER SIX

Dental Caries

Objectives

After completion of this chapter, the student will be able to:

▶ Define dental caries.

▶ Discuss dental caries in terms of progression, etiology and prevention.

▶ Discuss the clinical and radiographic examinations for caries.

▶ List the criteria for a diagnostic bite-wing film.

▶ Discuss how to interpret caries on a dental radiograph.

▶ List technique and exposure errors that affect interpretation of caries.

▶ Identify and describe the radiographic appearance of the following: incipient, moderate, advanced and severe interproximal dental caries.

▶ Identify and describe the radiographic appearance of the following: incipient, moderate and severe occlusal dental caries.

▶ Identify and describe the radiographic appearance of the following: buccal and lingual, root surface, recurrent and rampant caries.

▶ Define the terms *incipient* and *rampant*.

▶ List, describe and recognize the following conditions that may be confused with caries on a dental radiograph: restorative materials, abrasion, attrition and cervical burnout.

Key Words

Abrasion
Attrition
Bite-wing
Caries
Cavitation
Cervical Burnout
Contrast

Density
Incipient
Interpretation
Interproximal
Radiolucency
Rampant
Transillumination

Dental caries, or tooth decay, is one of the most common diseases that affects humans. Caries can be described as the localized destruction of teeth by microorganisms. Normal mineralized tooth structure is altered and destroyed by dental caries. As a result of the destruction, dental caries appears *radiolucent* on a radiograph. Dental caries is the most frequently encountered radiolucent lesion seen on dental radiographs.

Some carious lesions can be detected by simply looking in the mouth, others cannot. Interproximal lesions may be difficult, if not impossible, to detect clinically. Intraoral radiographs, such as the bite-wing, are indispensable in the detection of dental caries. Dental radiographs provide the dental health professional with essential diagnostic information concerning caries that cannot be derived from any other source. Caries detection is probably the most frequent reason for taking dental radiographs.

The purpose of this chapter is to review the description, detection, interpretation and radiographic classifications of dental caries as well as the conditions that are often confused with dental caries.

DESCRIPTION, DETECTION AND INTERPRETATION OF CARIES

In order to understand why caries appears radiolucent on a dental radiograph, an understanding of the caries process is necessary. The dental health professional must be familiar with the definition, description, progression, etiology and prevention of caries.

The dental professional must be able to detect dental caries both clinically and radiographically. Clinically, the practitioner must know how and where to look for caries. Any changes in tooth color and consistency must be carefully evaluated. The limitations of a clinical examination in the detection of interproximal caries must be recognized; some interproximal lesions can be detected clinically, others cannot. Understanding the importance of dental radiographs in the detection and diagnosis of interproximal dental caries is essential. The bite-wing, the dental radiograph of choice for the detection of caries, allows the dental professional to view the interproximal surfaces of the teeth. In order to adequately view the interproximal tooth surfaces on a bite-wing radiograph, the contact areas must be open (no overlapping) and the film must be of diagnostic quality.

In addition to knowing the basics about dental caries and caries detection, the clinician must be competent in the interpretation of dental caries as seen on a dental radiograph. The dental health professional needs to be familiar with the radiographic appearance of dental caries and the errors in technique and exposure that may affect the interpretation of films. Radiographs should always be evaluated with the patient present; any areas that appear to represent caries on a dental film should be verified clinically. If the patient is not present during the interpretation of dental films, important clinical information is lacking.

Caries Description

Definition

The term **caries** comes from the Latin *cariosus,* which means ''rottenness.'' Caries literally refers to rot of the teeth. Dental caries can be described as a destructive process that causes the decalcification of enamel followed by the destruction of enamel and dentin, and cavitation of a tooth. Caries is often referred to as tooth decay or a cavity in a tooth. In dentistry, the term *cavity* refers to a **cavitation,** or hole, seen in a tooth as the result of the caries process.

Progression

Caries left untreated progresses through the enamel and dentin and causes inflammation and death of the dental pulp. Caries that involves the dental pulp can cause intense pain until the pulp dies or is extirpated via endodontic therapy, or the tooth is extracted. Decayed teeth that involve the dental pulp may be a potential source of infection in the human body. Such teeth can interfere with the proper chewing of food, which can, in turn, lead to nutritional deficiencies and digestive disorders.

Etiology

Dental caries may occur in any area where plaque and food can adhere to the teeth. Certain bacteria found in the mouth break down sugars and starches and create an acid capable of destroying tooth enamel. In order for the caries process to occur, a number of variables must exist: bacteria that produce acid and cause decay, ingestion of foods that contribute to acid formation, inadequate plaque removal and host susceptibility factors, such as composition of teeth and saliva and ingestion of fluoride.

Prevention

At the present time, there is no cure for dental caries. Prevention appears to be the best approach to controlling this disease. Good oral hygiene, a diet limited in refined sugars and starches, fluoridated water and regular dental checkups all contribute to the prevention of dental caries.

Caries Detection

In order to detect dental caries, both a careful clinical examination and radiographic examination are necessary. A dental examination for caries cannot be considered complete without radiographs. The dental radiograph enables the dental professional not only to evaluate the extent and severity of a carious lesion seen clinically but also to identify carious lesions that are not visible clinically.

Clinical Examination

All teeth should be examined clinically for dental caries. The dental professional should have a set sequence for the caries examination. The examination should begin with tooth #1, followed by tooth #2, #3, etc., and end with tooth #32. All exposed and accessible surfaces should be examined for dental caries. All positive and suspicious clinical findings should be documented in the patient record and evaluated with dental radiographs.

In order to ensure good visibility, a bright operatory light should be used in the clinical examination. A mirror and explorer can be used to examine the teeth for evidence of dental caries. The mirror can be used to reflect light, to allow for indirect vision and to retract the tongue. The explorer can be used as a tactile device to detect the presence of any consistency changes (e.g., catches or tug-back) in the pits, fissures and grooves of the teeth.

Compressed air can be used to dry teeth and remove debris in order to allow for a better visual examination. A small flashlight can be used to detect dental caries on anterior teeth. **Transillumination,** or the passage of light through the tooth, allows the clinician to determine if the enamel is healthy. When the anterior teeth are illuminated with light, healthy areas of enamel permit the passage of the light, areas involved with caries do not.

Clinically, a number of color changes may be seen with dental caries. Occlusal surfaces may exhibit dark staining in the fissures, pits and grooves, or exhibit a gross, or obvious, cavitation. Smooth tooth surfaces may exhibit a chalky white spot or opacity indicating demineralization. An interproximal ridge overlying a carious lesion may appear discolored also.

A radiograph of any suspicious area that exhibits a change in consistency or color can give the practitioner additional information concerning the extent and severity of the lesion present. In some instances, no color change, cavitation or consistency changes are noted clinically. It is in these cases that radiographs play such an important role in the identification of dental caries.

Radiographic Examination

Radiographs are useful in the detection of caries because of the nature of the disease process. Demineralization and destruction of hard tooth structures result in a loss of tooth density in the area of the lesion. The decreased density allows a greater penetration of x-rays in the carious area, and as a result, the carious lesion appears as a **radiolucency** on a dental radiograph. As discussed in Chapter 2, radiolucent structures permit the passage of the x-ray beam and appear dark or black on a dental radiograph. The degree of radiolucency seen on a dental radiograph is determined by the extent and severity of the destruction seen as a result of the caries process.

Caries is *always* farther advanced clinically than what is seen on a dental radiograph. The early changes associated with demineralization do not affect the density of the tooth, and consequently, an increased penetration of the x-ray beam is not seen.

The **bite-wing** radiograph, a radiograph that shows the crowns of both the upper and lower teeth on the same film, is the radiograph of choice for the evaluation of dental caries. A periapical radiograph utilizing the paralleling technique can also be used to detect interproximal caries. In order for a bite-wing radiograph to be considered diagnostic for the evaluation of dental caries, the following criteria should be met:

- **Exposure and processing:** Proper film exposure and processing techniques must be used.
- **Open contacts:** Interproximal areas must demonstrate *open* contacts; a thin radiolucent line should be seen between the contacts of adjacent teeth (Fig. 6–1).
- **Occlusal plane:** The occlusal plane should be positioned horizontally along the midline of the long axis of the film (see Fig. 6–1).

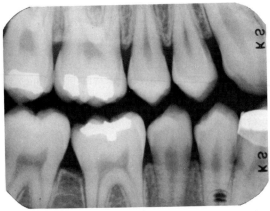

FIGURE 6–1. The open contacts in the premolar region appear as thin radiolucent lines. Note the occlusal plane is positioned horizontally along the midline of the long axis of the film.

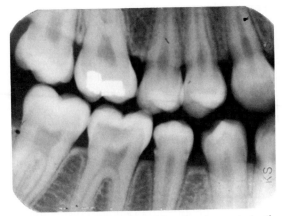

FIGURE 6–2. A good premolar bite-wing demonstrates the distal contact areas between the canine and first premolar.

- **Premolar placement:** The premolar bite-wing should demonstrate the distal contact areas of both the maxillary and mandibular canines (Fig. 6–2).
- **Molar placement:** The molar bite-wing should be centered over the second molar (Fig. 6–3).
- **Errors:** The bite-wing should be free of technique errors (e.g., cone cuts, film bending and backward film).

Caries Interpretation

Radiographic **interpretation,** or the ability to read what is revealed by a dental radiograph, is an important component of patient care. The dental hygienist can facilitate patient care by performing a preliminary radiographic interpretation. In order to play an important role in the interpretation of dental radiographs, the hygienist must be confident in the recognition of dental caries.

Interpretation Tips

As reviewed in Chapter 1, proper film mounting and viewing techniques are essential in the interpretation of dental radiographs, especially in the evaluation of dental caries. All films must be mounted before interpretation. An illuminator or viewbox is required to accurately view and interpret radiographs. If the screen of the viewbox is not completely covered by the mounted radiographs, the harsh light around the mounted films should be masked to reduce glare and intensify the detail and contrast of the radiographic images.

Films should be viewed in a room with subdued lighting that is free of distractions. The use of a pocket-sized magnifying glass is helpful in evaluating the radiographic appearance of dental caries and can be used to detect slight changes in density and contrast. Dental radiographs should always be interpreted with the patient present.

The dental professional should use a systematic approach to view and interpret films. Each time films are viewed, the same logical, step-by-step method should be used. Films should be viewed from left to right, just as you would read a printed page. Each tooth should be carefully examined from proximal surface to proximal surface and from the occlusal surface to the root apex. Interproximal caries is most likely to be seen *at* or *just below* (apical to) the contact area (Fig. 6–4). Interproximal caries and other types of dental caries that can be viewed on a dental radiograph are discussed in detail in this chapter.

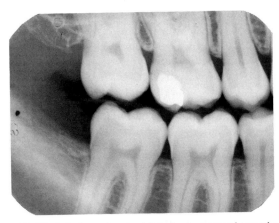

FIGURE 6–3. A good molar bite-wing is centered over the second molar.

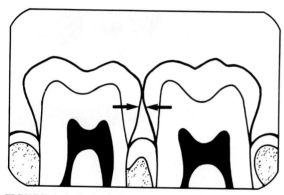

FIGURE 6–4. Caries is found at or just below the contact area.

Factors Influencing Caries Interpretation

A number of factors can influence the interpretation of dental caries as viewed on a dental radiograph. Radiographs must be of diagnostic quality in order to evaluate dental caries. Errors in technique and/or exposure may result in non-diagnostic films. Proper radiographic technique must be used. A bite-wing film used to detect dental caries must be free of overlapped contacts. Improper horizontal angulation causes overlapping of the contact areas of the crowns of the teeth and makes it impossible to interpret the interproximal regions for dental caries (Fig. 6–5).

Density and contrast are important in the detection of caries. **Density,** or the overall blackness of a film, is controlled by the milliamperage (mAs), kilovoltage (kVp) and exposure settings on a dental x-ray machine. Proper mAs, kVp and exposure time settings are necessary to produce a film with optimum density. Dental radio-

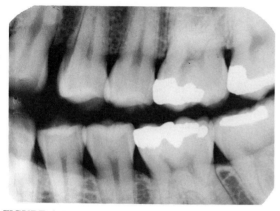

FIGURE 6–5. A nondiagnostic bite-wing with overlapped interproximal contacts.

graphs that are too dark or too light are useless in the detection of caries (Fig. 6–6).

Contrast refers to the difference in densities between adjacent areas on a dental film. Contrast is controlled by kVp. Kilovoltages between 65 and 70 produce a high-contrast film and are recommended for bite-wing films. Optimum contrast enhances caries detection.

The developing process affects both the density and contrast of dental radiographs. Precise developing time and fresh, clean developing solutions are necessary to produce films of diagnostic quality.

RADIOGRAPHIC CLASSIFICATION OF CARIES

The radiographic appearance of dental caries can be classified according to the location of the caries on the tooth. Caries involving the interproximal, occlusal, buccal, lingual and root surfaces may all be seen on a dental radiograph. In addition, recurrent and rampant caries may also be viewed on dental radiographs.

Interproximal Caries

Interproximal means "between two adjacent surfaces." Caries found between two teeth in the interproximal region can be viewed on a dental radiograph. Interproximal caries is typically seen at or just below (apical to) the contact point (Fig. 6–7). This area is difficult, if not impossible, to examine clinically. If the area could be examined clinically, the carious lesion would initially appear as a chalky white spot. As the demineralization process progresses, a roughness or stained area would be seen next, followed by cavitation. Three or four years may elapse before an interproximal lesion becomes clinically apparent.

As caries progresses inward through the enamel of the tooth, it assumes a triangular configuration; the apex (or point) of the triangle is seen at the dentino-enamel junction, or DEJ (Fig. 6–8). As a caries reaches the DEJ, it spreads laterally along the DEJ and continues into dentin. Another triangular configuration is seen in dentin, this time the base of the triangle is found along the DEJ and the apex is pointed toward the pulp chamber (Fig. 6–9). The triangular configuration of dental caries can be viewed on dental radiographs.

Interproximal caries can be classified accord-

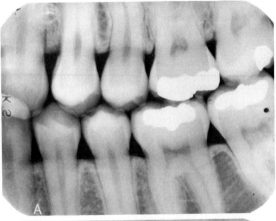

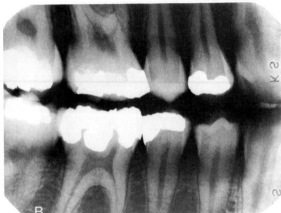

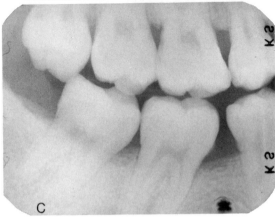

FIGURE 6–6. *A,* Diagnostic bite-wing radiograph. *B,* Nondiagnostic bite-wing radiograph (too dark). *C,* Nondiagnostic bite-wing radiograph (too light).

Incipient Interproximal Caries

The term **incipient** means ''beginning to exist or appear.'' An incipient lesion is a small carious lesion seen in enamel *only*. On a dental radiograph, an incipient, or Class I, lesion appears as a tiny radiolucent notch in the interproximal region (Fig. 6–10). An incipient interproximal le-

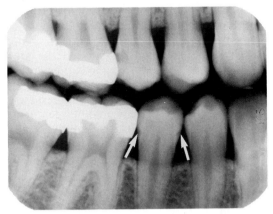

FIGURE 6–7. Interproximal caries is found at or just below the contact area.

ing to the depth of penetration the lesion exhibits through the enamel and dentin. Interproximal carious lesions viewed on a dental radiograph can be classified as incipient, moderate, advanced or severe.

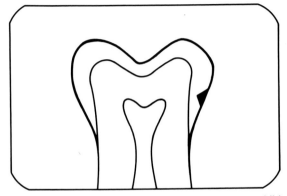

FIGURE 6–8. When confined to enamel, caries may exhibit a triangular configuration.

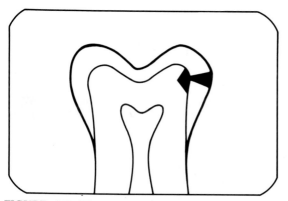

FIGURE 6–9. When caries reaches the dentino-enamel junction (DEJ), it spreads along the DEJ and another triangular configuration is seen.

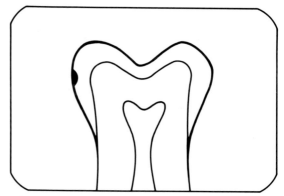

FIGURE 6–10. An incipient carious lesion extends less than halfway through the enamel.

sion is defined as one that extends less than halfway through the thickness of enamel (Fig. 6–11).

Moderate Interproximal Caries

A **moderate** interproximal lesion is defined as one that extends more than halfway through the thickness of enamel but does not involve the DEJ (Fig. 6–12). A moderate, or Class II, lesion is seen in enamel *only*. On a dental radiograph, a moderate interproximal lesion typically appears as a radiolucent triangle with the apex of the triangle near, but not involving, the DEJ (Fig. 6–13).

Advanced Interproximal Caries

An interproximal carious lesion that extends to the DEJ or through the DEJ and into dentin but does not extend through the dentin more than half the distance toward the pulp is termed **advanced** (Fig. 6–14). An advanced, or Class III, lesion affects *both* enamel and dentin. On a dental radiograph, an advanced interproximal lesion may appear as a triangular radiolucency in the enamel that reaches and involves the DEJ or as a large radiolucency that extends through the enamel and into the dentin but less than half the distance to the pulp (Figs. 6–15 and 6–16).

Severe Interproximal Caries

Caries that extends through the enamel and dentin and more than half the distance toward the pulp is termed **severe** (Fig. 6–17). Severe, or Class IV, interproximal caries involves *both* the enamel and dentin and is seen as a large radiolucency extending from the interproximal region

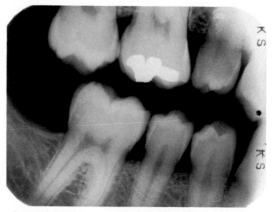

FIGURE 6–11. An incipient carious lesion is seen on the distal of the mandibular second premolar.

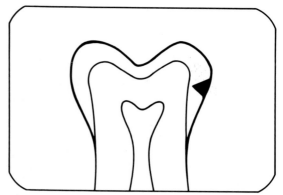

FIGURE 6–12. A moderate carious lesion extends greater than halfway through the enamel but does not involve the DEJ.

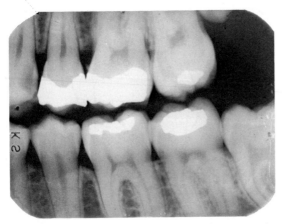

FIGURE 6–13. A moderate carious lesion is seen on the distal of the mandibular second premolar.

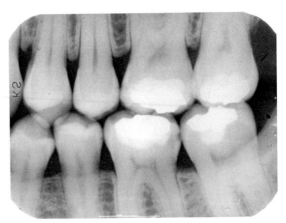

FIGURE 6–16. An advanced carious lesion that extends through the DEJ and into dentin is seen on the distal of the mandibular first molar.

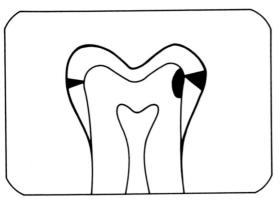

FIGURE 6–14. An advanced carious lesion extends through enamel and to or through the DEJ but does not extend through dentin greater than half the distance to the pulp chamber.

into the crown of a tooth (Fig. 6–18). Clinically, severe caries may appear as a hole or a cavity in the tooth (Fig. 6–19).

Occlusal Caries

Caries that involves the chewing surface of the posterior teeth is termed **occlusal.** A thorough clinical examination (as described earlier) using a mouth mirror and explorer is the method of choice for the detection of occlusal caries. Because of the superimposition of the dense buccal and lingual enamel cusps, early occlusal caries is difficult to see on a dental radiograph; consequently, occlusal caries is not seen on a radiograph until the DEJ is involved. Occlusal caries can be classified as incipient, moderate or severe.

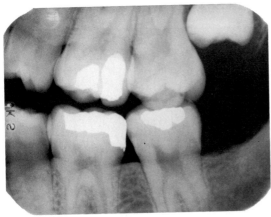

FIGURE 6–15. An advanced carious lesion that extends to the DEJ is seen on the mesial of the mandibular second molar.

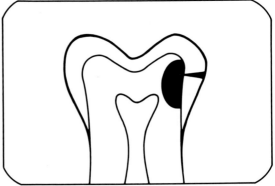

FIGURE 6–17. A severe carious lesion extends through enamel and dentin greater than half the distance to the pulp chamber.

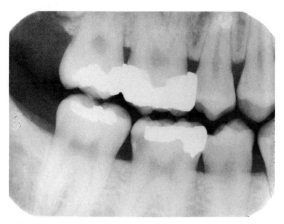

FIGURE 6–18. A severe carious lesion is seen on the distal of the mandibular first molar.

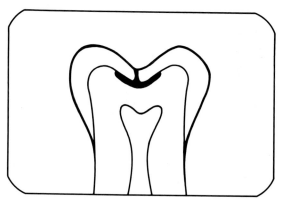

FIGURE 6–20. A moderate occlusal carious lesion extends through enamel and into dentin along the DEJ.

Incipient Occlusal Caries

Small incipient occlusal carious lesions cannot be seen on a dental radiograph and must be detected clinically instead.

Moderate Occlusal Caries

Moderate occlusal carious lesions may be seen as a very thin radiolucent line in dentin (Fig. 6–20). The thin radiolucency is located under the enamel of the occlusal surface of the tooth (Fig. 6–21). Little, if any, radiographic changes can be noted in the enamel. Once the DEJ is affected, the caries spreads laterally and then extends downward toward the pulp.

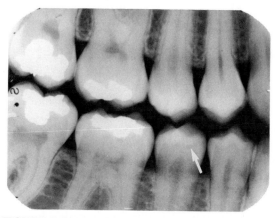

FIGURE 6–21. Occlusal caries is seen as a tiny radiolucency just below the DEJ on the mandibular second premolar.

Severe Occlusal Caries

Severe occlusal caries is seen as a large radiolucency in dentin (Figs. 6–22 and 6–23). Clini-

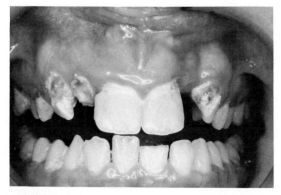

FIGURE 6–19. Severe caries may appear as a hole or cavity in a tooth. (Photo courtesy of Dr. Carl M. Allen, Associate Professor, Section of Diagnostic Services, The Ohio State University College of Dentistry.)

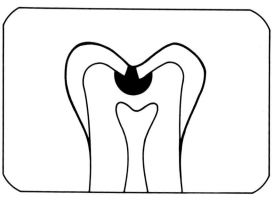

FIGURE 6–22. Severe occlusal caries extends through enamel and into dentin beyond the DEJ.

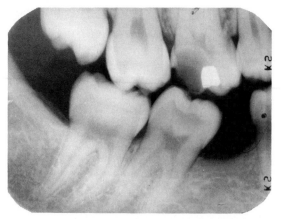

FIGURE 6–23. A severe occlusal carious lesion is seen as a large radiolucency in dentin on the mandibular first molar.

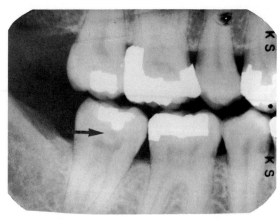

FIGURE 6–25. Buccal caries is seen as a small, circular radiolucency on the mandibular second molar.

cally, severe occlusal caries is apparent and appears as a hole, or *cavity,* in a tooth.

Buccal and Lingual Caries

Caries of the buccal and lingual surfaces of the teeth is best detected clinically. Because of the superimposition of the densities of normal tooth structure, buccal and lingual caries may be difficult to detect on a dental radiograph. When viewed on a dental radiograph, caries that involves the buccal or lingual surface appears as a small circular radiolucency (Figs. 6–24 and 6–25). If such a radiolucency is detected on a dental film, it is difficult to differentiate a buccal lesion from a lingual one. The radiolucency may appear better defined if the lesion is located on the lingual because of the close approximation of the film to the area of caries. In order to determine the location of the lesion, a clinical examination is necessary.

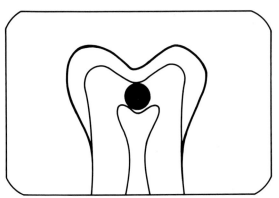

FIGURE 6–24. Buccal or lingual caries is seen as a round radiolucency on molars.

Root Surface Caries

As the name suggests, **root surface caries** involves the cementum and dentin of the roots of teeth, and occurs just below the cervical region of the tooth. No enamel is involved. Bone loss and corresponding gingival recession precede the caries process and result in exposed root surfaces. Plaque and debris accumulate in this area and lead to cervical root caries. A rapid penetration of caries through root dentin is not uncommon, and pulpal involvement is frequent.

Clinically, root surface caries can be easily seen on exposed root surfaces. The most common locations include the exposed roots of the mandibular premolar and molar areas. The buccal surfaces of the root are most frequently involved, followed by the lingual and proximal surfaces. Clinically, root caries appears saucer-shaped with a brownish color and leathery texture. On a dental radiograph, root caries appears as a cupped-out or crater-shaped radiolucency in the interproximal region just below the cemento-enamel junction, or CEJ (Figs. 6–26 and 6–27). Early lesions may be difficult to detect on a dental radiograph.

Recurrent Caries

Recurrent, or secondary, caries is seen adjacent to a preexisting restoration. Caries occurs in this region because of inadequate cavity preparation, defective margins or incomplete removal of caries before the placement of a restoration. On a dental radiograph, recurrent caries appears as a radiolucent area just beneath a restoration (Fig. 6–28). Recurrent caries is most often seen

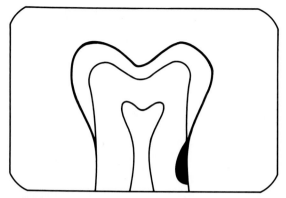

FIGURE 6–26. Root caries involves cementum and dentin only, *not* enamel.

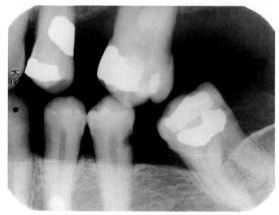

FIGURE 6–27. Root caries appears as a crater-shaped radiolucency just below the cemento-enamel junction (CEJ) on the mandibular second premolar.

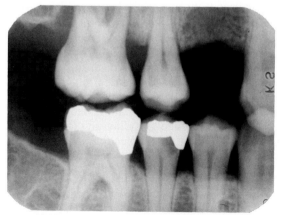

FIGURE 6–28. Recurrent caries is seen as a radiolucency below a two-surface amalgam restoration on the mandibular second premolar.

beneath the interproximal margins of a restoration.

Rampant Caries

The term **rampant** means growing or spreading unchecked and refers to advanced and severe caries that affects numerous teeth in the dentition (Fig. 6–29). Rampant caries may be seen in children with poor dietary habits or in adults with a decreased salivary flow.

CONDITIONS RESEMBLING CARIES

A number of radiolucencies that involve the crown and roots of teeth are seen on a dental radiograph and may be confused with dental caries. Restorative materials, abrasion, attrition and cervical burnout may all resemble dental caries on a radiograph. The dental professional must remember that the final diagnosis of caries is made only after the clinical and radiographic findings are corroborated. Both the clinical examination and interpretation of radiographs are mutually contributory aids in making the diagnosis of dental caries.

Restorative Materials

Restorative materials, such as composites, silicates and acrylics, may appear radiolucent and resemble dental caries on a radiograph (see Chapter 5). The appearance of anterior cavity preparations restored with these materials differs from the appearance of interproximal decay (Fig. 6–30) and can be identified by its well-defined, smooth outlines (Fig. 6–31). In addition, a careful clinical exam helps the dental professional in determining the difference between a restorative material and dental caries.

Abrasion

Abrasion refers to the wearing away of tooth structure from the friction of a foreign object. The surface of the tooth affected depends on the causative factor. The most frequent type of abrasion is caused by tooth brushing and is seen at the cervical margin of the teeth. Tooth brush abrasion affects the root surface of a tooth and may be confused with root surface caries. On a dental radiograph, tooth brush abrasion appears

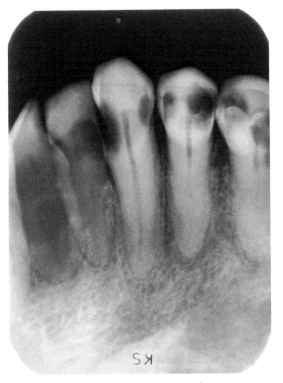

FIGURE 6–29. Rampant caries.

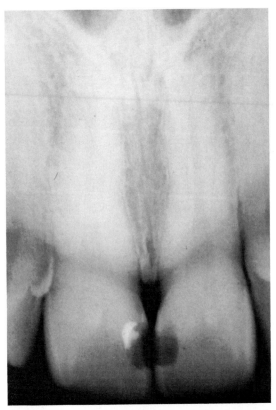

FIGURE 6–31. Anterior composite restorations have well-defined smooth outlines.

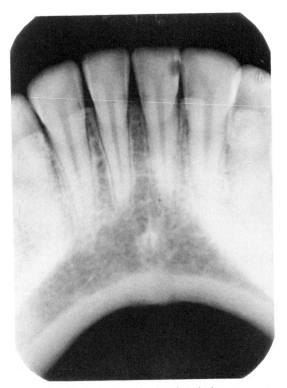

FIGURE 6–30. An interproximal carious lesion seen on an anterior tooth appears as an ill-defined radiolucent area.

as a well-defined horizontal radiolucency along the cervical region of a tooth (Fig. 6–32). Clinically, the areas affected by abrasion appear as hard, highly polished defects in dentin and should not be confused with root caries, which appears brown and leathery.

Attrition

Attrition, or the mechanical wearing down of teeth, may be mistaken for dental caries on a radiograph. Attrition may be seen on the incisal or occlusal surfaces of deciduous or permanent teeth. When the incisal or occlusal enamel is worn away, the underlying dentin wears away rapidly, and shallow concavities may form. These concavities may resemble occlusal or incisal caries on a dental radiograph (Fig. 6–33). Clinical examination enables the dental professional to distinguish attrition from caries.

Cervical Burnout

Cervical burnout, a radiolucent artifact seen on dental radiographs, may also be confused with

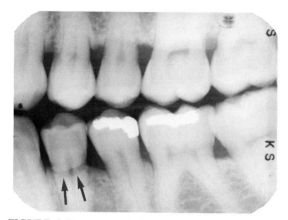

FIGURE 6–32. Toothbrush abrasion appears as a radiolucent area around the CEJ.

dental caries. Cervical burnout appears as a collar or wedge-shaped radiolucency on the mesial and distal root surfaces near the CEJ of a tooth. When seen as a radiolucent collar (Fig. 6–34), cervical burnout may be confused with root caries. This radiolucent artifact is seen because of the difference in densities of adjacent tissues. The tissue density at the cervical region of the tooth is less dense than the regions above and

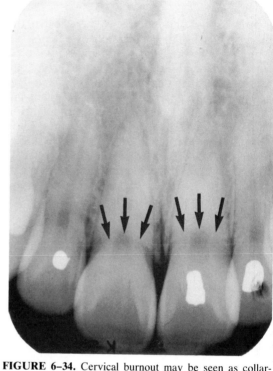

FIGURE 6–34. Cervical burnout may be seen as collar-shaped radiolucent areas.

below it; above the neck of the tooth, enamel covers the crown, and below the neck of the tooth, bone covers the roots.

Cervical burnout can also appear as an ill-defined wedge-shaped radiolucency on the mesial or distal root surfaces near the CEJ of posterior teeth (Fig. 6–35). This wedge-shaped radiolucency is seen because of the anatomic root concavities found in this area.

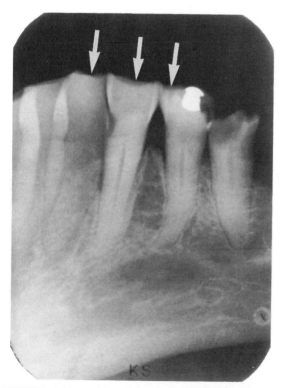

FIGURE 6–33. Attrition occurs on the occlusal and incisal surfaces of teeth and appears as a radiolucent area.

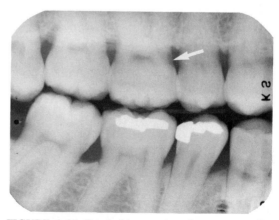

FIGURE 6–35. Cervical burnout may be seen as wedge-shaped radiolucent areas.

SUMMARY

Dental caries, or tooth decay, is a destructive process causing decalcification of enamel, destruction of enamel and dentin and cavitation of teeth. Dental caries can be detected through the use of a thorough clinical examination and diagnostic radiographs. Both a clinical exam and radiographs are necessary to make a diagnosis. Clinically, the dental professional must know how and where to look for dental caries and be familiar with the radiographic appearance of caries. On a dental radiograph, caries appears radiolucent. Of all the radiolucent lesions that can be found on dental radiographs, dental caries is seen most frequently.

Dental caries may involve any surface of the tooth crown or root. Caries seen on a dental radiograph may be classified as interproximal, occlusal, buccal or lingual or those involving the root surfaces. Caries may also be seen as a recurrent lesion under an existing restoration or as a rampant problem, affecting many teeth in the dentition. Dental caries may be mistaken for a number of other radiolucencies, including restorative materials, abrasion, attrition and cervical burnout.

Bibliography

DeLyre WR and Johnson ON: Preliminary interpretation of the radiographs. *In* Essentials of Dental Radiography for Dental Assistants and Hygienists, pp 181–83. Norwalk, CT: Appleton and Lange, 1990.

Frommer HH: Radiographic interpretation: caries, periodontal disease, and pulpal, peripical, and bone lesions. *In* Radiology for Dental Auxiliaries, pp 275–83. St. Louis: CV Mosby, 1987.

Goaz PW and White SC: Dental caries. *In* Cook DB (ed.): Oral Radiology Principles and Interpretation, 2d ed., pp 381–401. St. Louis: CV Mosby, 1987.

Langland OE, Sippy FH and Langlais RP: Radiologic interpretation of dental disease. *In* Textbook of Dental Radiography, 2d ed., pp 432–51. Springfield, IL: Charles C Thomas, 1984.

Miles DA, et al.: Interpretation: normal versus abnormal. *In* Radiographic Imaging for Dental Auxiliaries, pp 202–7. Philadelphia: WB Saunders, 1989.

QUIZ QUESTIONS

"What Can This Be?"

For questions 1 to 8, identify the carious lesion (location and severity) or the condition the radiolucency represents.

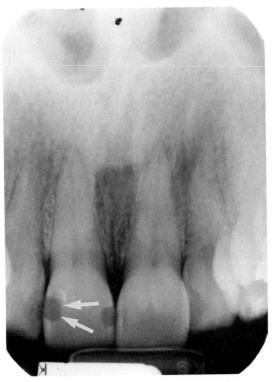

1.

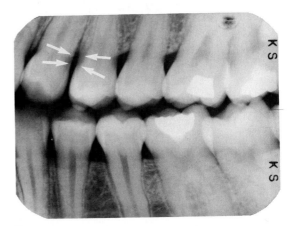

2.

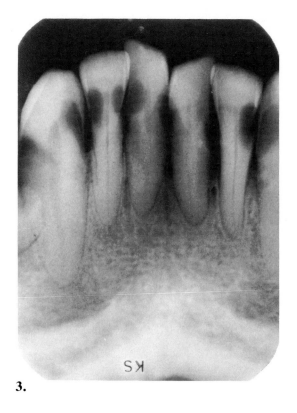

3.

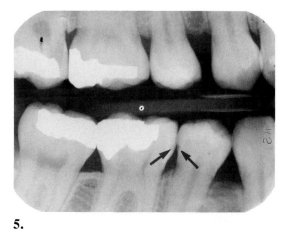

5.

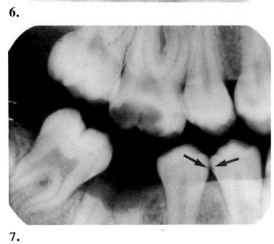

6.

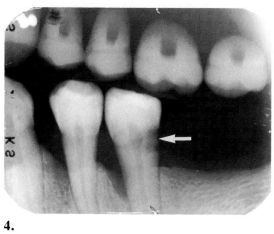

4.

7.

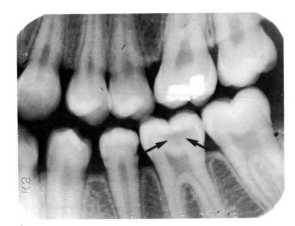

8.

Matching

For questions 9 to 16, match the classification of radiographic caries with the appropriate description.

_____ **9.** Incipient interproximal

A. An interproximal carious lesion that extends more than halfway through the enamel but does not involve the DEJ.

_____ **10.** Moderate interproximal

B. An interproximal carious lesion that extends to the DEJ or through the DEJ but does not extend more than half the distance through dentin toward the pulp chamber.

_____ **11.** Advanced interproximal

C. An interproximal lesion that extends through enamel, through dentin and more than half the distance toward the pulp.

_____ **12.** Severe interproximal

D. An interproximal lesion that extends less than halfway through enamel.

_____ **13.** Incipient occlusal

E. Seen as a large radiolucency in dentin; a large hole may be seen clinically on the chewing surface of the tooth.

_____ **14.** Moderate occlusal

F. Appears as a thin radiolucent line below occlusal enamel on a dental radiograph.

_____ **15.** Severe occlusal

G. Cannot be seen on a radiograph.

For questions 16 to 20, match the terms on the left with the appropriate definition.

_____ **16.** Incipient

A. Mechanical wearing down of teeth.

_____ **17.** Rampant

B. Wearing away of tooth structure from friction of a foreign object.

_____ **18.** Attrition

C. Spreading unchecked.

_____ **19.** Cervical burnout

D. Radiolucent artifact.

_____ **20.** Abrasion

E. Beginning to exist or appear.

CHAPTER SEVEN

Periodontal Disease

Objectives

After completion of this chapter, the student will be able to:

▶ Define the terms *periodontium* and *periodontal*.

▶ Define the healthy periodontium (soft tissue and bone).

▶ Define periodontal disease.

▶ Discuss the importance of dental radiographs in the diagnosis of periodontal disease.

▶ List and describe the type of radiographs that should be used to document periodontal disease and the preferred exposure technique.

▶ Discuss the limitations of radiographs in the diagnosis of periodontal disease.

▶ Define the terms *generalized, localized, horizontal bone loss, vertical bone loss* and *furcation involvement*.

▶ Define each of the four ADA Case Types and describe the corresponding radiographic appearance.

▶ Recognize each of the four ADA Case Types on dental radiographs.

▶ List the predisposing factors for periodontal disease.

▶ Recognize and describe the radiographic appearance of calculus.

▶ Define, describe and recognize a periodontal abscess as it appears on a radiograph.

Key Words

ADA Case Types
Alveolar crest
Calculus, subgingival
Calculus, supragingival
Cemento-enamel junction
Furcation involvement
Generalized bone loss
Gingivitis
Horizontal bone loss

Lamina dura
Localized bone loss
Periodontal
Periodontal abscess
Periodontal disease
Periodontal ligament space
Periodontitis
Periodontium
Stippled
Vertical bone loss

Dental radiographs play an integral role in the assessment of periodontal disease. A radiographic examination is essential for diagnostic purposes and enables the practitioner to obtain vital information concerning supporting bone that cannot be obtained clinically. In order to make the diagnosis of periodontal disease, both a clinical examination and radiographs are necessary. Dental radiographs are an adjunct to the clinical examination, not a substitute for it. Dental radiographs serve to detect changes in bone, approximate the amount and location of bone loss, identify predisposing factors and aid in the evaluation and prognosis of affected teeth.

This chapter describes the healthy periodontium and periodontal disease and discusses the clinical and radiographic detection of periodontal disease. The importance and limitations of dental radiographs are presented as well. Also included in this chapter is the radiographic interpretation of periodontal disease with emphasis on description of bone loss, ADA Case Types and identification of predisposing factors.

RECOGNITION OF PERIODONTAL DISEASE

The Healthy Periodontium

In order to recognize periodontal disease, the dental professional must first be familiar with the clinical appearance of healthy gingival tissue and the radiographic appearance of normal alveolar bone. The term **periodontium** refers to tissues that invest and support the teeth, such as the gingiva and alveolar bone. Healthy gingival tissue is generally described as coral pink, although the color may vary depending on the individual's race. The consistency of healthy gingiva is firm and resilient, and the interproximal margins are knife-edged as they closely adapt to the teeth. Clinically, healthy gingiva exhibits no bleeding upon instrumentation and minimal sulcus depth upon probing. The gingiva appears **stippled** in texture and resembles the surface of an orange peel.

The radiographic appearance of normal alveolar bone has been previously described in Chapter 3. The normal anatomic landmarks of alveolar bone include the **lamina dura, alveolar crest** and **periodontal ligament space.** In health, the lamina dura around the roots of the teeth appears as a dense, radiopaque line (Fig. 7–1). The normal healthy alveolar crest is located approximately 1.5 to 2.0 mm apical to the

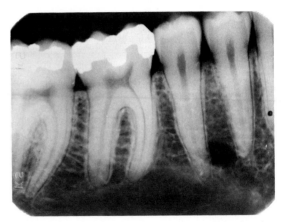

FIGURE 7–1. Healthy alveolar crest, normal lamina dura and periodontal ligament space seen on a periapical radiograph.

cemento-enamel junctions (CEJ) of adjacent teeth.

The shape and density of the alveolar crest vary between the anterior and posterior regions of the mouth. In the anterior regions, the alveolar crest appears pointed and sharp and is normally very radiopaque (Fig. 7–2). In the posterior regions, the alveolar crest appears flat, smooth, and parallel to a line between adjacent cemento-enamel junctions (Fig. 7–3). The al-

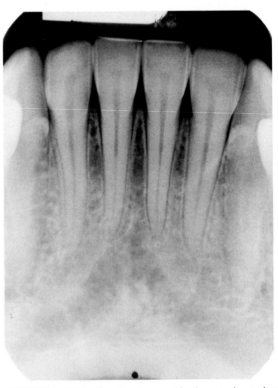

FIGURE 7–2. Healthy alveolar crest in the anterior region appears pointed and very radiopaque.

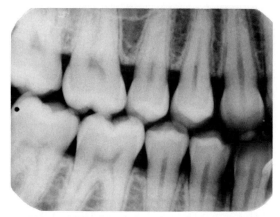

FIGURE 7–3. Healthy alveolar crest in the posterior region appears flat, smooth and radiopaque.

veolar crest in the posterior regions appears a bit less radiopaque than in the anterior regions.

The normal periodontal ligament space appears as a thin radiolucent line between the root of the tooth and the lamina dura. In health, the periodontal ligament space is continuous around the root structure and of uniform thickness (see Fig. 7–1).

Description of Periodontal Disease

The term **periodontal** literally means "around a tooth." **Periodontal disease** refers to a group of diseases that affect the tissues around the teeth. Periodontal disease may range from a superficial inflammation of gingiva **(gingivitis)** to the destruction of the supporting bone and periodontal ligament **(periodontitis).** With periodontal disease, the gingiva exhibits varying degrees of inflammation. The gingival tissues affected by periodontal disease do not appear stippled, firm and pink. Instead, the gingiva appears swollen, red and bleeding, and pocket formation is seen. The radiographic appearance of alveolar bone affected by periodontal disease differs from that of healthy alveolar bone. The alveolar crest is no longer located 1.5 to 2.0 mm apical to the cemento-enamel junctions and no longer appears radiopaque. Periodontal disease may result in the severe destruction of bone and the loss of teeth.

DETECTION OF PERIODONTAL DISEASE

In order to detect periodontal disease, both clinical and radiographic examinations are neces-

sary. Dental radiographs *must* be used in conjunction with a clinical exam. In general, what is seen clinically cannot be evaluated on dental radiographs, and what is viewed on dental radiographs cannot be evaluated clinically. The clinical exam provides information about soft tissue while radiographs permit the evaluation of bone.

Clinical Examination

The clinical exam should include an evaluation of the gingival tissues for signs of inflammation, such as redness, bleeding, swelling, rounded gingival margins and purulent exudate. Changes within gingival tissues can best be detected by periodontal probing. A thorough periodontal assessment should not only include periodontal probing but a gingival index and evaluation of the attached gingiva as well. With advanced disease, mobility and furcation charting is necessary. Whenever there is clinical evidence of disease, radiographs must be taken in order to obtain maximum diagnostic information. All clinical findings should be adequately documented in the patient record.

Radiographic Examination

Radiographs, along with a clinical exam, allow the dental professional to diagnose, evaluate and determine the prognosis of periodontal disease. The radiographic examination supplements the clinical examination. The extent of alveolar bone loss can best be determined by radiographs. Dental radiographs provide important information concerning the supporting bone that cannot be seen clinically. Crestal changes, bone loss, changes in the width and shape of the periodontal ligament space and furcation involvements can all be viewed on dental radiographs. Just as all clinical findings concerning periodontal disease must be recorded in the patient record, all radiographic findings must be documented as well.

RADIOGRAPHS AND PERIODONTAL DISEASE

Importance of Radiographs

Dental radiographs provide an overview of the amount of bone present and indicate the pattern, distribution and severity of bone loss that has taken place as a result of periodontal disease. Radiographs can be used to evaluate the condition of the crestal bone, lamina dura, periodontal ligament space, length and structure of tooth roots and any furcation involvements present. Dental radiographs can also be used to identify predisposing factors and aid in the evaluation and prognosis of affected teeth.

Radiographs allow the dental professional to document periodontal disease. Dental radiographs serve as a permanent record of the condition of a patient's bone at a specific point in time. Initial radiographs documenting periodontal disease can be used as a baseline; all subsequent follow-up radiographs can then be compared with the baseline films to determine the success or failure of periodontal therapy.

Types of Radiographs

The periapical film is the film of choice for evaluating periodontal disease. While the horizontal bite-wing radiograph has limited use in the detection of periodontal disease, the vertical bite-wing can be used as a post-treatment film. The panoramic film is not recommended for the evaluation of periodontal disease.

Periapical Films

Periapical dental radiographs are recommended for the patient with periodontal disease. A periapical film shows the entire crown and root of a tooth along with alveolar bone (Fig. 7–4). This film allows for optimal evaluation of the supporting bone. Periapicals should be exposed with a kVp of 75 to 100 in order to penetrate structures adequately and allow visualization of bony details.

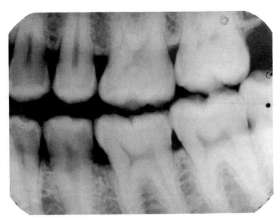

FIGURE 7–5. A bite-wing radiograph shows early changes in bone.

Bite-Wing Films

The horizontal bite-wing radiograph can be used to detect interproximal calculus and early to moderate bony changes seen with periodontal disease (Fig. 7–5). Severe interproximal bone loss cannot be adequately visualized on horizontal bite-wing radiographs (Fig. 7–6). The vertical bite-wing radiograph can be used to examine bone levels throughout the mouth (Fig. 7–7). The vertical bite-wing is useful as a post-treatment or follow-up film for periodontal maintenance patients. When compared with a complete series of periapicals (14 or 15 films), less films are used with a vertical bite-wing exam (a total of seven).

Panoramic Films

The panoramic radiograph has little diagnostic value in the identification of periodontal disease and is *not* recommended to demonstrate the an-

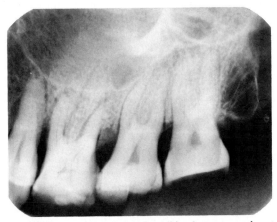

FIGURE 7–4. A periapical film exhibits the crown and root of a tooth along with supporting bone.

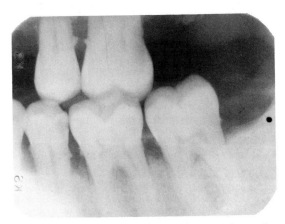

FIGURE 7–6. A bite-wing radiograph cannot be used to document moderate to severe bone loss.

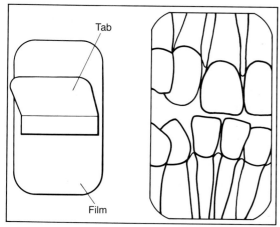

FIGURE 7–7. A vertical bite-wing can be used to evaluate the level of supporting bone.

atomic features of the condition. Although the panoramic radiograph shows the clinician a single continuous view of the bone supporting the teeth, there is a marked lack of definition of dental structures, and the interproximal bone and periodontal ligament space cannot be adequately visualized (Fig. 7–8).

Radiographic Technique Preferred

The long-cone paralleling technique is the preferred method of exposure for periapical films used to demonstrate the anatomic features of periodontal disease. With the long-cone paralleling technique, the height of crestal bone is accurately recorded in relation to the tooth root. If the bisection-of-the-angle technique is used to expose periapical radiographs, a dimensional distortion of bone is seen because of the vertical angulation used. As a result, periapicals using the bisection-of-the-angle technique may appear to show more or less bone loss than is actually present (Figs. 7–9 and 7–10). Also with the bisection-of-the-angle technique, calculus may be superimposed on alveolar bone and may not be detected on the radiographs.

Limitations of Radiographs

There are a number of limitations to the use of dental radiographs in the detection and diagnosis of periodontal disease. Radiographs alone cannot be used to diagnose periodontal disease; they must be used in conjunction with a thorough clinical examination. Dental radiographs do not provide information concerning the condition of soft tissue or the existence of soft tissue pockets. In addition, dental radiographs do not record the early bony changes seen with periodontal disease.

Because dental radiographs record two-dimensional images of three-dimensional structures, certain areas of teeth and bone are difficult, if not impossible, to examine radiographically. Buccal and lingual areas are particularly difficult to evaluate. Bone loss in furcation areas may not be detected on a dental radiograph because of the superimposition of buccal and lingual bone. Calculus located on buccal or lingual surfaces of teeth may be difficult to detect, and bony or osseous defects overlapped by existing bony walls may also be overlooked on a dental radiograph.

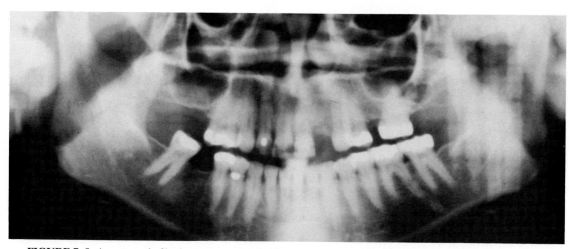

FIGURE 7–8. A panoramic film is not recommended for the evaluation and documentation of periodontal disease.

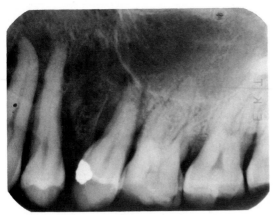

FIGURE 7–9. Because of the vertical angulation used, bisection-of-the-angle technique may distort the level of bone present.

Radiographs and Treatment Evaluation

The use of follow-up serial radiographs can be used in determining the success of periodontal treatment. In order to compare pre-treatment and post-treatment radiographs, the radiographs must be standardized in terms of film placement, angulation of the beam, exposure factors and processing techniques. Post-treatment radiographs indicating successful periodontal therapy exhibit no additional bone loss. Lack of evidence of additional bone loss over a period of time suggests that the disease is arrested or quiescent. The cortical bone in interseptal areas may appear more radiopaque on post-treatment films. Post-treatment radiographs should not exhibit features indicative of an active, destructive process but rather a static condition.

RADIOGRAPHIC INTERPRETATION OF PERIODONTAL DISEASE

In addition to identifying periodontal disease clinically, the dental professional must be competent in the interpretation of periodontal disease as viewed on dental radiographs. The practitioner must be familiar with the radiographic appearance of periodontal disease. Radiographs should be evaluated for crestal irregularities, interseptal alveolar bone changes, pattern, distribution and severity of bone loss, furcation involvements and the presence of local irritants or predisposing factors. All radiographic findings should be documented in the patient record.

Bone Loss

A dental radiograph allows the dental professional to view the amount of bone remaining rather than the amount of bone lost. However, in documenting bone levels, the amount of bone loss that has occurred is recorded versus the amount of bone that remains. The amount of bone loss can be estimated as the difference between the physiologic bone level and the height of remaining bone (Fig. 7–11). Bone loss can best be evaluated with dental radiographs and must be described in the patient record according to the pattern, distribution and severity of loss.

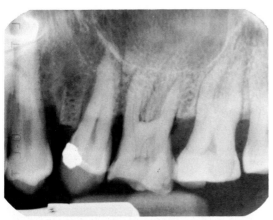

FIGURE 7–10. Paralleling technique used to examine the same area seen in Figure 7–9. Note the difference in bone level. With the paralleling technique, the height of crestal bone is accurately recorded in relation to the tooth root.

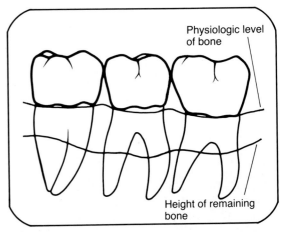

Physiologic level of bone

Height of remaining bone

FIGURE 7–11. Bone loss is estimated as the difference between the physiologic level of bone and the height of remaining bone.

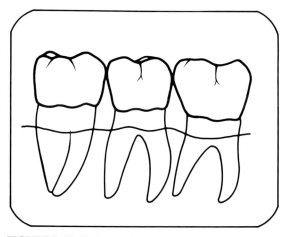

FIGURE 7–12. Horizontal bone loss occurs in a plane parallel to the cemento-enamel junctions of adjacent teeth.

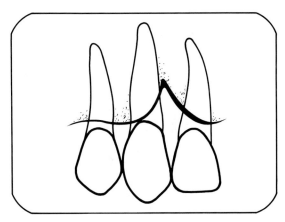

FIGURE 7–14. Vertical bone loss occurs in a plane that is not parallel to the cemento-enamel junctions of adjacent teeth.

Pattern

The pattern of bone loss viewed on a dental radiograph can be described as either *horizontal* or *vertical*. The cemento-enamel junctions of adjacent teeth can be used as a plane of reference in determining the pattern of bone loss present. With **horizontal bone loss,** the bone loss occurs in a plane parallel to the cemento-enamel junctions of adjacent teeth (Figs. 7–12 and 7–13). Horizontal bone loss appears to lower the height of alveolar bone. **Vertical bone loss,** also known as angular bone loss, does not occur in a plane parallel to the cemento-enamel junctions of adjacent teeth (Figs. 7–14 and 7–15).

Distribution

The distribution of bone loss viewed on a dental radiograph can be described as *localized* or *gen-*

eralized, depending on the number of areas of interseptal bone involved. **Localized bone loss** occurs in isolated areas (Fig. 7–16). **Generalized bone loss** occurs evenly throughout the dental arches (Fig. 7–17). The distribution of bone loss is important in treatment decisions and prognosis.

Severity

The extent of bone loss viewed on a dental radiograph can be classified as either *mild, moderate* or *severe*. Bone loss is measured on a dental radiograph as a percentage loss of the normal amount of bone. Normal alveolar bone height spans from the apex of a tooth to a point approximately 1.5 to 2.0 mm below the CEJ of the tooth. A transparent template can be used to assist the dental professional in estimating the

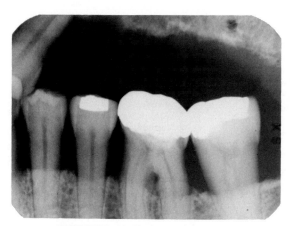

FIGURE 7–13. Horizontal bone loss.

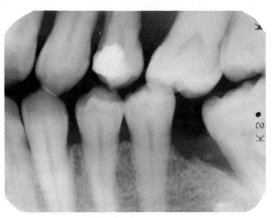

FIGURE 7–15. Vertical bone loss.

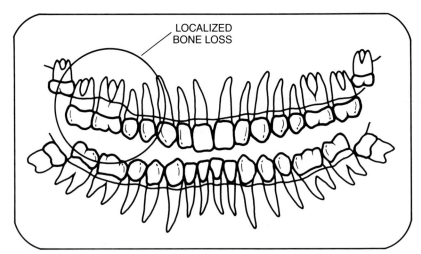

FIGURE 7–16. Localized bone loss occurs in isolated areas.

amount of bone loss viewed on a dental radiograph (Fig. 7–18). Mild bone loss can be described as a loss of approximately 20% to 30% (Fig. 7–19), moderate as a 30% to 50% loss (Fig. 7–20), and severe as a 50% or more loss (Fig. 7–21).

Classification of Periodontal Disease

In addition to describing the bone loss viewed on dental radiographs in terms of pattern, distribution and severity, periodontal disease can be classified according to the clinical and radiographic findings. The American Academy of Periodontology has categorized periodontal disease into four categories: **ADA Case Type I** (gingivitis), **ADA Case Type II** (early periodontitis), **ADA Case Type III** (moderate periodontitis) and **ADA Case Type IV** (advanced periodontitis).

ADA Case Type I

Type I disease is known as *gingivitis* or the inflammation of the gingiva resulting from the presence of bacterial plaque. Gingivitis from local irritation is the earliest form of periodontal disease. With gingivitis, the gingiva clinically appears reddened and inflamed. Bleeding upon instrumentation and slight pocket formation are present. There is *no* bone loss associated with gingivitis, and therefore, *no* radiographic change in the bone is seen.

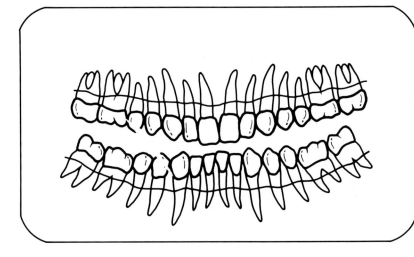

FIGURE 7–17. Generalized bone loss occurs throughout the dental arches.

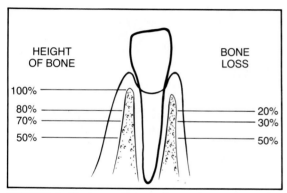

FIGURE 7–18. A template can be used to estimate the amount of bone loss viewed on a dental radiograph.

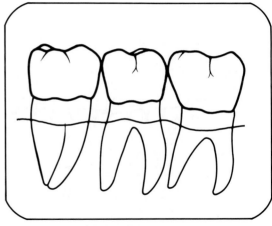

FIGURE 7–20. Moderate bone loss.

ADA Case Type II

If gingival inflammation is permitted to persist and progresses to involve the alveolar bone, *early periodontitis,* or Type II disease, results. Clinically, early periodontitis exhibits all or some of the signs of gingivitis, and redness, bleeding, swelling and exudation may be seen. In addition, pocket formation is identified clinically.

Radiographically, early changes in the alveolar bone are seen as an indistinct fuzziness of the crestal lamina dura. The bone loss associated with early periodontitis can be viewed on a dental radiograph and described as mild to moderate (approximately 20% to 30%) (Figs. 7–22 and 7–23).

ADA Case Type III

Type III disease, or *moderate periodontitis,* is seen with further destruction of the periodon-

tium. Clinically, the signs of inflammation previously described for Type I and Type II disease are seen with moderate periodontitis. In addition, moderate to deep pockets are visible.

Bone loss is described as moderate to severe (30% to 50%) and can be readily detected on dental radiographs (Figs. 7–24 and 7–25). The pattern of bone loss may be horizontal or vertical; the distribution may be localized or generalized. **Furcation involvement,** or the extension of periodontal disease between the roots of multi-rooted teeth, may also be seen with Type III disease. When the bone in the furcation area is destroyed, a radiolucent area is evident on the dental radiograph (Fig. 7–26). Tooth mobility and osseous defects may also be seen.

ADA Case Type IV

Advanced periodontitis, or Type IV disease, occurs when bone loss is so extensive that the

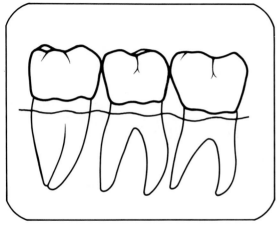

FIGURE 7–19. Mild bone loss.

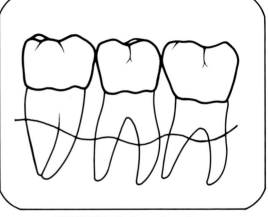

FIGURE 7–21. Severe bone loss.

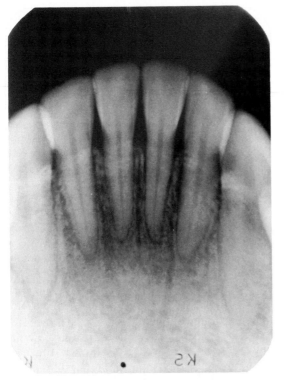

FIGURE 7–22. ADA Case Type II.

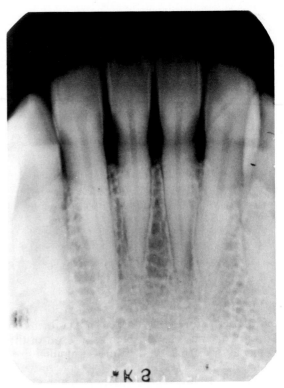

FIGURE 7–24. ADA Case Type III.

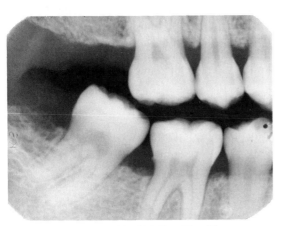

FIGURE 7–23. ADA Case Type II.

Predisposing Factors

A number of predisposing factors or local irritants contribute to periodontal disease. The identification, detection and elimination of local irritants are important in the management and treatment of periodontal disease. Dental radiographs play a major role in the detection of local irritants, such as calculus and defective restorations.

teeth show excessive mobility from the lack of bony support. The progressive destruction of the supporting structures seen in Type IV disease often results in the loss of teeth. With Type IV disease, a severe destruction of periodontal structures is seen along with severe bone loss, tooth mobility and furcation involvement. Bone loss is described as over 50% (Figs. 7–27 and 7–28).

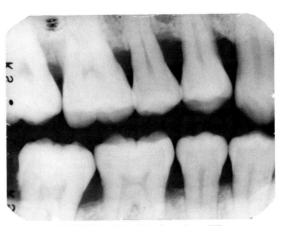

FIGURE 7–25. ADA Case Type III.

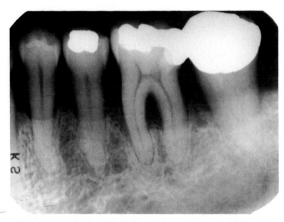

FIGURE 7–26. The furcation area of the mandibular first molar appears radiolucent.

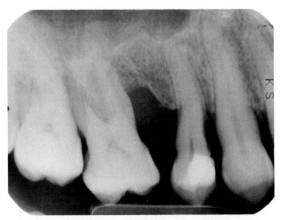

FIGURE 7–28. ADA Case Type IV.

Calculus

Calculus is a stone-like concretion that forms on the crowns and roots of teeth as a result of the calcification of bacterial plaque. Calculus prevents the cleansing of the gingival sulcus, acts as a local irritant to adjacent gingival tissues and is a contributing or predisposing factor to periodontal disease.

Calculus may be found above or below the gingival margin and may or may not be detected on a dental radiograph. **Supragingival calculus** (calculus found above the gingiva) is most often located on the lingual surfaces of the mandibular anterior teeth or the buccal surfaces of the maxillary molars. When viewed on a dental radiograph, calculus found in these areas is superimposed over the crowns of the teeth and may be difficult, or impossible, to detect (Fig. 7–29).

Subgingival calculus (calculus found below the

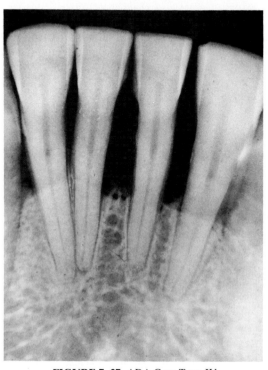

FIGURE 7–27. ADA Case Type IV.

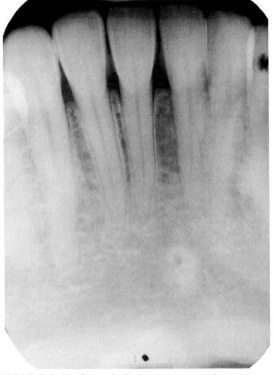

FIGURE 7–29. Supragingival calculus seen in the interproximal areas of the mandibular anterior region.

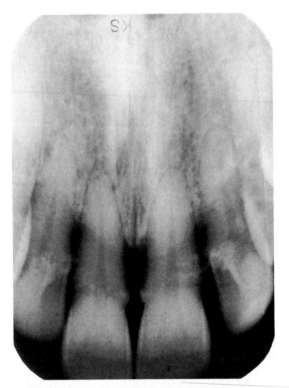

FIGURE 7–30. Subgingival calculus seen as irregular radiopaque projections in the maxillary anterior region.

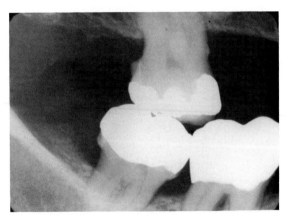

FIGURE 7–32. Calculus may appear as a ring-like radiopacity around the cervical region of a tooth.

radiopaque projection (Fig. 7–33) or a smooth radiopacity on a root surface (Fig. 7–34).

Defective Restorations

Faulty dental restorations act as potential food traps and lead to the accumulation of food debris and bacterial deposits. Trapped debris and bacteria damage soft tissue and lead to inflam-

gingiva) can be easily detected and appears radiopaque on a dental radiograph (Fig. 7–30). Although subgingival calculus may exhibit a variety of appearances on a dental radiograph, it most often appears as pointed or irregular radiopaque projections extending from proximal root surfaces (Fig. 7–31). Calculus may also appear as a ring-like radiopacity encircling the cervical portion of a tooth (Fig. 7–32), a nodular

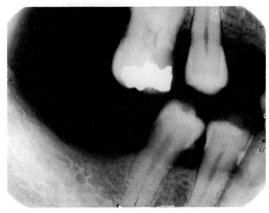

FIGURE 7–31. Calculus may appear as sharp pointed radiopacities.

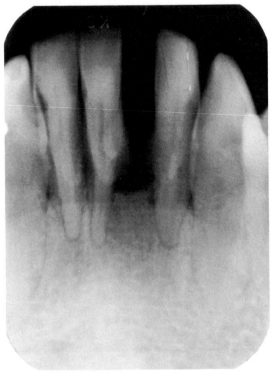

FIGURE 7–33. Calculus may appear nodular as seen here between two mandibular incisors.

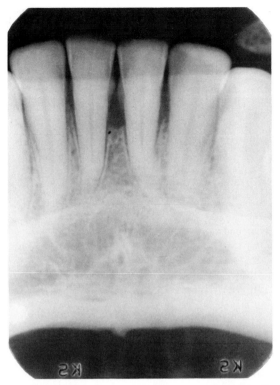

FIGURE 7–34. Calculus may appear as a smooth radiopacity.

mation and periodontal disease. Defective restorations can be detected both clinically and radiographically. Radiographs allow the dental professional to identify restorations with open or loose contacts (Fig. 7–35), poor contour (Fig. 7–36), uneven marginal ridges (Fig. 7–37), overhangs (Fig. 7–38) and shy margins (Fig. 7–39), all of which may contribute to periodontal disease.

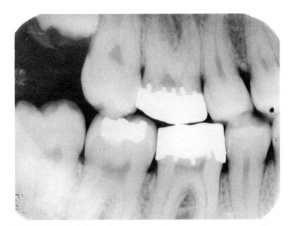

FIGURE 7–36. Poorly contoured crowns seen on maxillary and mandibular first molars.

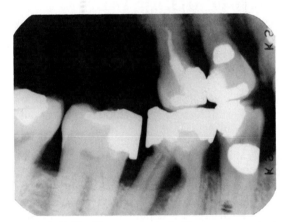

FIGURE 7–37. Uneven marginal ridges, open contact, overhangs, and poorly contoured restorations seen on this bite-wing radiograph.

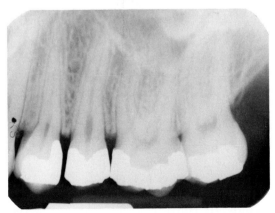

FIGURE 7–35. Open contact seen between maxillary premolars.

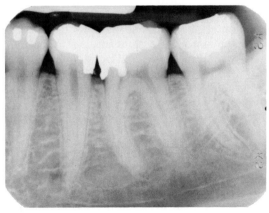

FIGURE 7–38. Amalgam overhang seen on the mesial of the mandibular first molar.

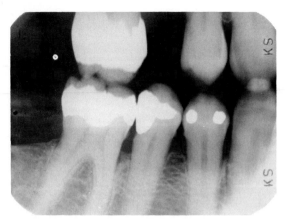

FIGURE 7–39. Shy margin seen on distal of mandibular second premolar.

CONDITIONS ASSOCIATED WITH PERIODONTAL DISEASE

There are several conditions associated with periodontal disease that may be detected on a dental radiograph. The dental radiograph plays an important role in diagnosing periodontal abscesses and identifying occlusal trauma and tooth mobility.

Periodontal Abscess

A **periodontal abscess** can be described as a destructive lesion that originates in a soft tissue pocket. A localized collection of pus forms as a result of the invasion of pyogenic bacteria seen secondary to the partial or complete occlusion of a soft tissue pocket. Drainage of pus may occur around the neck of the tooth or via a sinus tract in alveolar bone. Entrapment of foreign bodies (e.g., popcorn husks, seeds or toothbrush bristles) can initiate the formation of a periodontal abscess. The periodontal abscess has potential to cause rapid and extensive bone loss. Several millimeters of periodontal attachment and alveolar bone can be destroyed in a matter of days.

Periapical radiographs and vitality testing are necessary to diagnose a periodontal abscess. The periodontal abscess is not a pulpal problem, and therefore, the tooth pulp should test vital. On a dental radiograph, a periodontal abscess appears as a radiolucency around the root surface of a tooth. In severe cases, bony destruction can be so extensive that no bone is seen around the roots, and the tooth appears to be floating (Fig. 7–40).

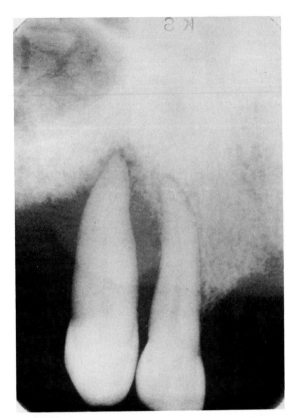

FIGURE 7–40. Extensive destruction of bone seen in association with a periodontal abscess.

Mobility

Mobility of teeth can be caused by injury of the supporting structures of the teeth. Tooth mobility cannot always be detected on a dental radiograph. A widened periodontal ligament space is a radiographic indication of tooth mobility and the result of resorption of both the root and alveolar bone (Fig. 7–41).

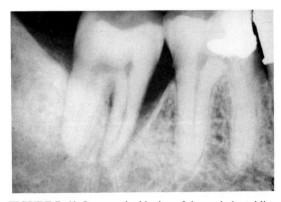

FIGURE 7–41. Increased widening of the periodontal ligament space seen on the mesial of the mandibular second molar. Clinically, this tooth exhibits mobility.

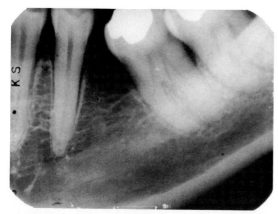

FIGURE 7–42. Increased widening of the periodontal ligament space is seen around the mandibular second premolar as a result of occlusal trauma.

Occlusal Trauma

As a result of occlusal trauma, the bony wall of the tooth socket and periodontal ligament space may undergo varying changes. Occlusal trauma may involve one tooth, several teeth or the entire dentition.

Occlusal trauma occurs when excessive force is placed on a tooth as a result of premature contact. It is not uncommon for the patient suffering from occlusal trauma to complain of discomfort. The classic radiographic appearance of occlusal trauma is a widened periodontal ligament space (Fig. 7–42). Other radiographic changes that may be seen include decreased definition of the lamina dura, bone loss and altered trabecular patterns.

SUMMARY

Dental radiographs play a vital role in the detection, evaluation and diagnosis of periodontal disease. Both a thorough clinical and radiographic examination are necessary in order to make a diagnosis of periodontal disease. The clinical examination allows the practitioner to obtain information concerning soft tissue, while the radiographic examination provides information about the supporting bone. Radiographs allow the dental professional to document periodontal disease and determine the success or failure of therapy.

The dental professional must be competent in the interpretation of periodontal disease as viewed on dental radiographs. The interpretation of periodontal disease on radiographs should include an evaluation of crestal and interseptal alveolar bone. Any bone changes or bone loss should be described in terms of pattern, distribution and severity. Furcation involvements, presence of local irritants, periodontal abscesses or radiographic indications of mobility or occlusal trauma should be noted as well. All radiographic findings concerning periodontal disease should be documented in the patient record.

Bibliography

Carranza FA: Radiographs and other aids in the diagnosis of periodontal disease. *In* Glickman's Clinical Periodontology, 7th ed., pp 501–16. Philadelphia: WB Saunders, 1990.

Goaz PW and White SC: Periodontal disease. *In* Oral Radiology Principles and Interpretation, 2d ed., pp 406–18. St Louis: CV Mosby, 1987.

Grant DA, Stern IB and Everett FG: Periodontal health and disease. *In* Periodontics, 5th ed., pp 3–19. St. Louis: CV Mosby, 1979.

Langland OE, Sippy FH and Langlais RP: Radiologic interpretation of dental disease: periodontal disease. *In* Textbook of Dental Radiography, 2d ed., pp 476–501. Springfield, IL: Charles C Thomas, 1984.

Manson-Hing LR: Interpretation and value of radiographs. *In* Fundamentals of Dental Radiography, 3d ed., p 207. Philadelphia: Lea and Febiger, 1990.

Regezi JA and Sciubba JJ: Inflammatory jaw lesions. *In* Oral Pathology: Clinical-Pathologic Correlations, pp 393–94. Philadelphia: WB Saunders, 1989.

Sheridan PJ: Periodontal disease. *In* Gibilisco JA, ed., Stafne's Oral Radiographic Diagnosis, pp 94–110. Philadelphia: WB Saunders, 1985.

Wilkins EM: The gingiva. *In* Clinical Practice of the Dental Hygienist, 5th ed., pp 185–99. Philadelphia: Lea and Febiger, 1983.

QUIZ QUESTIONS

"What Can This Be?"

For questions 1 to 8, identify the pattern and severity of bone loss, and the ADA Case Type represented by each radiograph.

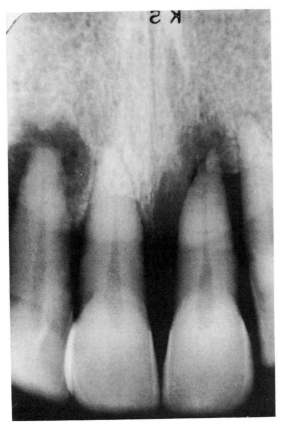

3.

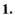

1.

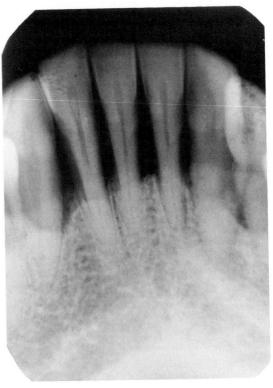

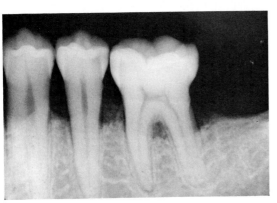

2.

4.

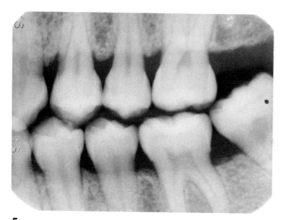

5.

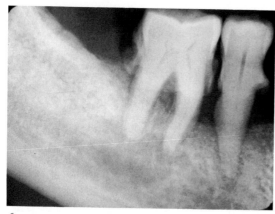

6.

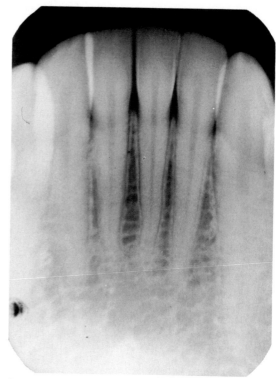

8.

Matching

For questions 9 to 12, match each of the ADA Case Types with the appropriate radiographic description.

_____ **9.** ADA Case Type I

_____ **10.** ADA Case Type II

_____ **11.** ADA Case Type III

_____ **12.** ADA Case Type IV

A. Mild to moderate bone loss (up to 20% to 30%).

B. Severe bone loss (more than 50%).

C. No bony change seen.

D. Moderate to severe bone loss (30% to 50%).

Fill In

For questions 13 to 21, fill in the blank.

13. _____ is a term that refers to tissues that invest and support the teeth.

14. _____ is a term that means "around a tooth."

15. _____ is a term that refers to the extension of periodontal disease between the roots of multirooted teeth.

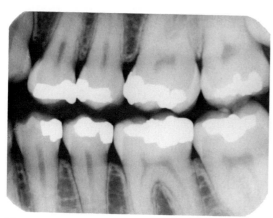

7.

16. _____ is the film of choice for the evaluation of periodontal disease.

17. _____ is the preferred method of exposure for films documenting periodontal disease.

18. _____ is a term that describes bone loss which occurs in a plane parallel to the cemento-enamel junctions of adjacent teeth.

19. _____ is a term that describes bone loss which does not occur in a plane parallel to the cemento-enamel junctions of adjacent teeth.

20. _____ is a term that refers to inflammation of the gingiva.

21. _____ is a term that describes a collection of pus that forms in a soft tissue pocket as a result of the occlusion of the pocket opening.

For questions 22 to 23, describe each of the following as radiolucent or radiopaque.

22. Calculus appears _____ on a dental radiograph.

23. A periodontal abscess appears _____ on a dental radiograph.

For questions 24 and 25, list two presdisposing factors to periodontal problems.

24. _____

25. _____

CHAPTER EIGHT

Trauma, Pulpal and Periapical Lesions

Objectives

After completion of this chapter, the student will be able to:

▶ Identify crown, root and jaw fractures as seen on dental radiographs.

▶ Define the terms *luxation, intrusion, extrusion* and *avulsion*.

▶ Identify intrusion, extrusion and avulsion as viewed on dental radiographs.

▶ Identify pulp chambers of normal, atrophic and enlarged sizes as viewed on dental radiographs.

▶ Identify pulp stones and obliteration of the pulp chamber as viewed on dental radiographs.

▶ Identify and describe a periapical radiolucency as viewed on a dental radiograph.

▶ Identify condensing osteitis, sclerotic bone and hypercementosis as viewed on a dental radiograph.

▶ Identify internal and external resorption as viewed on a dental radiograph.

Key Words

Avulsion
Condensing osteitis
External resorption
Extrusion
Fracture
Hypercementosis
Internal resorption
Intrusion
Luxation
Pathologic resorption

Periapical abscess
Periapical cyst
Periapical granuloma
Physiologic resorption
Pulp stones
Pulpal obliteration
Pulpal sclerosis
Sclerotic bone
Trauma

The dental radiograph is an indispensable diagnostic tool. In many instances, the dental radiograph is a detector and shows change. Changes from trauma and resorption can be easily viewed on dental radiographs as well as changes that affect the pulpal and periapical tissues of the teeth. The radiograph provides the dental health professional with essential diagnostic information concerning these changes that cannot be derived from any other source. The dental radiograph allows the practitioner to evaluate areas that cannot be examined clinically, such as the roots, pulp chambers and periapical regions of the teeth.

The dental professional must be competent in identifying changes associated with trauma and pulpal and periapical lesions viewed on dental radiographs. Each change or lesion identified on a dental radiograph must be documented in the patient record in terms of appearance, location and size. This chapter provides the reader with a review of the common radiographic features of change that affect the teeth and/or surrounding bone. Radiographic changes seen with trauma and resorption are presented along with the radiographic features of common pulpal and periapical lesions.

RADIOGRAPHIC CHANGES DUE TO TRAUMA

Trauma can be defined as an injury produced by an external force. Trauma may affect the crowns and roots of teeth as well as alveolar bone. Trauma may result in fractures of teeth and bone and injuries such as intrusion, extrusion and avulsion. Dental radiographs are important in evaluating the effects of trauma in the orofacial region. Radiographs are not only used to identify injuries but are useful in determining the location, orientation and degree of separation of fractures. With trauma, the radiograph is a valuable adjunct to the patient history and clinical examination. Radiographs are not only useful in the diagnostic process but in subsequent examinations as well. Post-treatment radiographs are often used to evaluate injured areas and screen for changes that may occur as a result of the trauma.

Fractures

A **fracture** can be defined as the breaking of a part. Fractures may affect the crowns and roots of teeth, or bones of the maxilla and mandible.

Whenever a fracture is evident or suspected, radiographic examination of the injured area is necessary. Dental radiographs can be used to diagnose fractures and to evaluate fractures for treatment and post-treatment purposes. Radiographic examination after trauma is helpful in monitoring the fracture site during repair.

Crown Fractures

Fractures that affect tooth crowns are most often seen in the anterior regions of the maxilla and mandible. Most crown fractures are seen as a result of an accident involving a fall or a vehicle. Crown fractures may involve the enamel only, the enamel and dentin, or the enamel, dentin and pulp.

Clinical Features. Clinically, a fracture that involves the enamel and dentin appears as a missing portion of the crown (Fig. 8–1). If the pulp chamber is involved, bleeding may be evident. Endodontic therapy is indicated when there is pulpal exposure or necrosis.

Radiographic Features. The missing part of a crown caused by a fracture is evident on a periapical radiograph (Fig. 8–2). The radiograph allows the dental professional to evaluate the proximity of the pulp chamber to the fracture and to examine the root for any additional fractures.

Root Fractures

Root fractures are less common than crown fractures. As with crown fractures, fractures of the root are seen as a result of an accident or traumatic blow. Root fractures occur most often in the maxillary central incisor region. Tooth

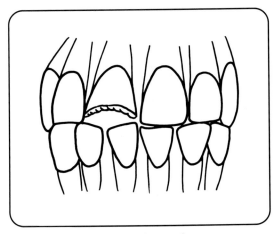

FIGURE 8–1. A fractured crown.

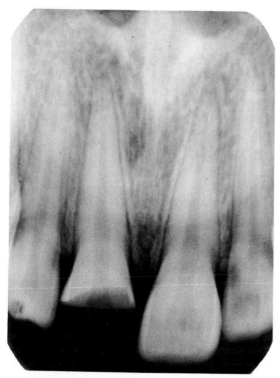

FIGURE 8-2. A fractured central incisor.

roots may be fractured at any level along the root and may involve more than one root of a multirooted tooth.

Clinical Features. A root fracture cannot be seen clinically. Excessive crown mobility, which can be detected clinically, suggests a root fracture. Crown mobility varies depending on the fracture location; the closer the root fracture is to the apex of the tooth, the more stable the crown. A tooth with a root fracture close to the apex has a good prognosis. If the root fracture occurs close to the crown, the prognosis is poor and extraction is indicated.

A tooth with a root fracture typically exhibits partial or complete sensitivity loss; however, in most cases, the sensitivity returns with time. Endodontic therapy is indicated when pulpal necrosis is seen as a result of the root fracture.

Radiographic Features. If the x-ray beam is parallel with the plane of the fracture, the root fracture appears as a sharp radiolucent line on a periapical radiograph (Fig. 8-3). If the x-ray beam is not parallel with the fracture, adjacent areas of tooth structure are superimposed over the fracture, and an ill-defined gray shadow is seen. Superimposition of surrounding alveolar bone may also cause difficulty in viewing a root fracture on a dental radiograph.

With time, root fractures have a tendency to enlarge from displacement of root fragments, hemorrhage or edema. Consequently, a root fracture initially overlooked may be identified on a later dental radiograph (Fig. 8-4). Oblitera-

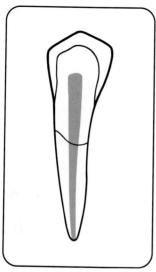

FIGURE 8-3. A fractured root.

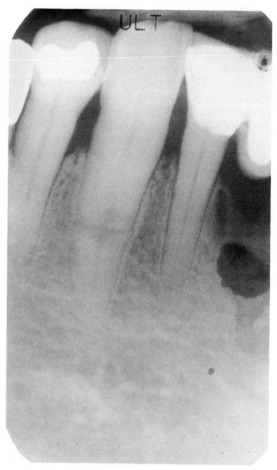

FIGURE 8-4. A root fracture seen on a mandibular canine.

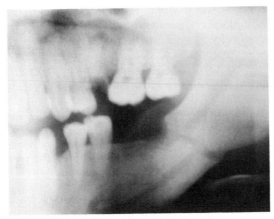

FIGURE 8–5. A fractured mandible.

tion of the pulp chamber resulting from a root fracture may also be seen with time.

Fractures of the Mandible

The mandible is fractured more often than any other bone of the face. Fractures of the mandible may include the body, ramus or condyles. Mandibular fractures frequently occur as the result of assaults, accidents and sports injuries and are often seen in association with injuries to other bones of the face and skull.

Clinical Features. A history of trauma along with facial swelling and pain is the typical presentation of a mandibular fracture. Manipulation of the mandible typically reveals abnormal mobility. Most mandibular fractures are treated with reduction, fixation or immobilization.

Radiographic Features. The panoramic radiograph is useful in the evaluation of mandibular fractures. Radiographically, a mandibular fracture appears as a radiolucent line at the site where the bone has separated (Figs. 8–5 and 8–6). In some cases, the bone at the fracture site overlaps and appears radiopaque along the margins of the fracture.

Fractures of the Maxilla

Anterior alveolar fractures are the most common fractures of the maxilla. Most maxillary alveolar injuries involve teeth and are seen secondary to trauma. Fractures of the midface may involve the maxilla alone or occur in conjunction with fractures of other bones found in the region.

Clinical Features. Anterior teeth are usually involved in alveolar fractures of the maxilla. The labial plate of alveolar bone is fractured more often than the palatal plate. With an anterior alveolar fracture, the fracture line usually occurs in a horizontal direction. Clinically, a patient with a maxillary alveolar fracture exhibits excessive mobility of the anterior segment along with a malocclusion. Treatment for a maxillary alveolar fracture includes the repositioning of displaced teeth and splint stabilization. Endodontic therapy may be required for the teeth involved.

Midface fractures are complex and can be classified as zygomatic complex, horizontal, pyramidal and craniofacial disjunction fractures. The clinical features and treatments vary depending on the type and severity of the fracture.

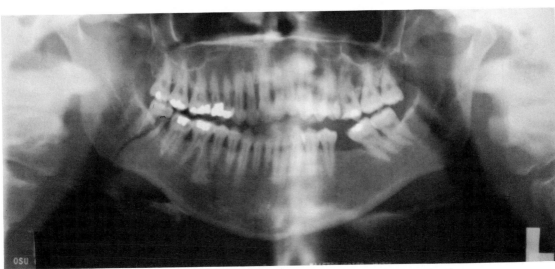

FIGURE 8–6. A fractured mandible that involves the mandibular second molar.

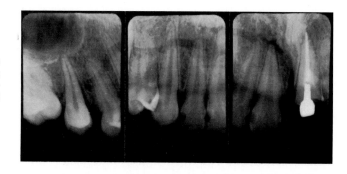

FIGURE 8–7. Maxillary alveolar process fracture as evidenced by radiolucent line. (Reproduced with permission from Gibilisco JA: Stafne's Oral Radiographic Diagnosis, 5th ed., p 357. Philadelphia: WB Saunders, 1985.)

Radiographic Features. When an alveolar fracture affects only the labial or palatal plates of the maxilla, the fracture is difficult to identify on an intraoral radiograph. However, a fracture of the maxilla that includes both the labial *and* palatal plates can usually be seen as a radiolucent line on an intraoral or extraoral radiograph (Fig. 8–7).

Radiographic examination of the midface region is often difficult because of the superimpositions of multiple anatomic structures. Films such as the posteroanterior, Waters's, reverse-Towne's, lateral skull and submentovertex may be utilized to view and identify fractures of the midface.

Injuries

Besides fractures, trauma may result in displacement of teeth. Injuries may include partial displacement of teeth into bone and partial or total displacement of teeth out of bone. Radiographs allow the dental professional to evaluate dental structures after injuries that cause displacement of teeth. A dental radiograph taken at the time of tooth displacement can be used to demonstrate the extent of root, periodontal ligament and alveolar bone injury. Radiographs taken at the time of injury can also be used as a reference for comparison with subsequent radiographs.

Luxation

Luxation can be defined as abnormal displacement of teeth. Abnormal displacement of teeth can be categorized as either intrusion or extrusion. **Intrusion** refers to the abnormal displacement of teeth *into* bone; **extrusion** refers to the abnormal displacement of teeth *out* of bone.

Clinical Features. A tooth that has been intruded or extruded is apparent clinically. The clinical crown of an intruded tooth appears shorter than the adjacent teeth (Fig. 8–8). In some instances, the entire crown may be displaced into the alveolar bone, in which case the crown is not apparent clinically and appears to be "lost." The clinical crown of an extruded tooth appears longer than adjacent teeth (Fig. 8–9).

Intrusion and extrusion are most likely to in-

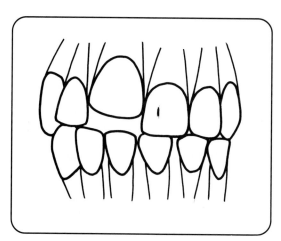

FIGURE 8–8. An intruded crown.

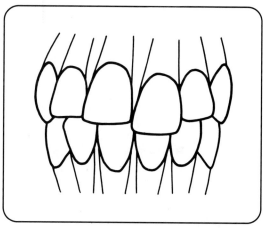

FIGURE 8–9. An extruded crown.

volve maxillary central incisors. As with all tooth movement associated with trauma, intrusion and extrusion have the potential to disrupt periapical circulation and induce temporary or permanent pulpal changes. Pulpal necrosis may take place as a result of intrusion or extrusion. In cases of pulpal necrosis, endodontic therapy is indicated.

Radiographic Features. Teeth that have been luxated should be evaluated with a periapical radiograph. The traumatized tooth must be examined for root and adjacent alveolar bone fractures, damage to the periodontal ligament and pulpal problems. A radiograph taken at the time of injury can be compared to subsequent radiographs for regressive alterations of the teeth that may take place.

Avulsion

Avulsion can be defined as the complete displacement of a tooth from alveolar bone. Most avulsions are seen as a result of trauma associated with an assault or accidental fall.

Clinical Features. A tooth that has been avulsed is apparent clinically since it is missing from the alveolar arch. Treatment may include reimplantation of the tooth, depending on the extent and severity of damage to the tooth and socket. The success of reimplantation depends on the time elapsed since avulsion and the vitality of the residual periodontal ligament fibers. The sooner the reimplantation of the tooth takes place, the better the prognosis. Endodontic therapy is indicated following the reimplantation of an avulsed tooth.

Radiographic Features. An avulsed tooth

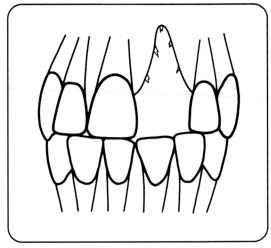

FIGURE 8–11. Splintered bone may be seen in a tooth socket.

is not seen on a radiograph. A periapical radiograph shows a tooth socket without a tooth (Fig. 8–10). Dental radiographs are important in the evaluation of the socket area and should be used to examine the region for splintered bone (Fig. 8–11). In addition, subsequent radiographs can be used to monitor the replacement of damaged bone, which may take months or years to fill in the socket area. In cases of reimplanted avulsed teeth, external resorption may be observed on radiographs.

RADIOGRAPHIC CHANGES DUE TO RESORPTION

Two types of resorption are seen with teeth: physiologic and pathologic. **Physiologic resorption** is a process that is seen with the normal shedding of primary teeth. The roots of a deciduous tooth are resorbed as the permanent successor moves in an occlusal direction (Fig. 8–12). The deciduous tooth is shed when resorption of the roots are complete. **Pathologic resorption** is resorption of teeth *not* associated with the normal shedding of deciduous teeth.

Pathologic resorption is a regressive alteration of tooth structure observed when a tooth is subjected to abnormal stimuli. Resorption of tooth surfaces may be seen as a result of chronic inflammation, abnormal pressure, external forces or idiopathic causes. Resorption of teeth can be described as external or internal, depending on the location of the resorption process. External and internal resorption have characteristic radiographic appearances.

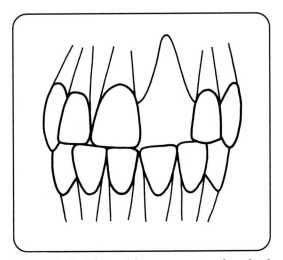

FIGURE 8–10. With avulsion, an empty tooth socket is seen on a dental radiograph.

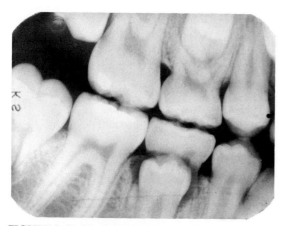

FIGURE 8–12. Physiologic resorption of a mandibular deciduous second molar.

External Resorption

External resorption takes place along the periphery of the root surface (Fig. 8–13). It is often associated with reimplanted teeth, abnormal mechanical forces, trauma, chronic inflammation, tumors, cysts, impacted teeth or idiopathic causes. External resorption is believed to be initiated by the destruction of the cementum or periodontal ligament along the root surface. External resorption may involve one or more teeth. Although any tooth may be involved, the anterior teeth are more frequently affected than posterior.

Clinical Features. External resorption is not associated with any signs or symptoms and therefore cannot be detected clinically. Teeth that undergo external resorption do not exhibit

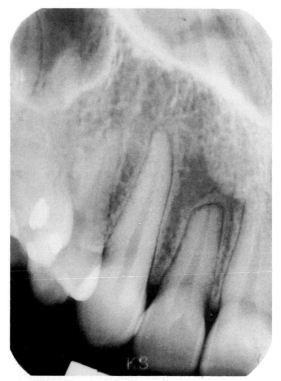

FIGURE 8–14. External resorption of the apical region of a maxillary lateral incisor.

mobility. There is no effective treatment for external resorption.

Radiographic Features. External resorption of root surfaces is readily identified on dental radiographs. External resorption most often affects the apices of teeth. As a result of the smooth resorption of root structure, the apical region appears blunted, and the length of the root appears shorter than normal (Figs. 8–14 and 8–15). Both the lamina dura and bone

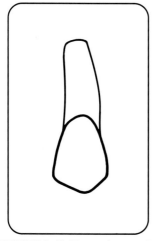

FIGURE 8–13. External resorption.

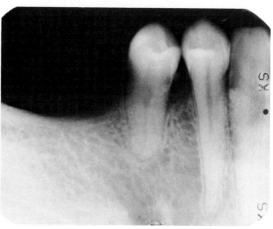

FIGURE 8–15. External resorption of a mandibular second premolar.

around the blunted apex appear normal. Occasionally, lateral root surfaces may undergo external resorption, in which case resorption of the lateral root surfaces may appear irregular rather than smooth.

Internal Resorption

Internal resorption occurs within the crown or root of a tooth and involves the pulp chamber, pulp canals and surrounding dentin (Fig. 8–16). Resorption of dentin surrounding pulp walls may be seen as a result of pulpal inflammation, or it may be seen in cases where no identifying factor can be determined. Several precipitating factors, including trauma, pulp capping and pulp polyps, have been suspected in the stimulation of the internal resorption process. Any tooth may be affected by internal resorption, and usually a single tooth is involved.

Clinical Features. Most cases of internal resorption are not apparent clinically. If internal resorption occurs within the crown of a tooth, the crown may exhibit a pinkish hue because of the close proximity of the pulp tissue to the tooth surface. Internal resorption is generally asymptomatic. Symptoms may occur if the lesion occurs in the root of the tooth; extensive resorption may weaken the root and a fracture may result.

Treatment for teeth affected by internal resorption is variable. If the resorptive process has not physically weakened the tooth and per-

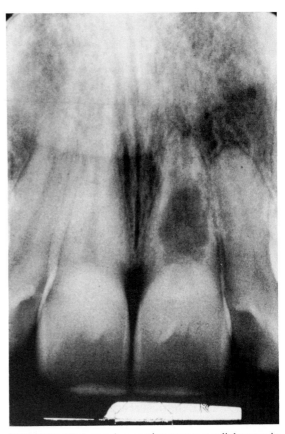

FIGURE 8–17. Internal resorption seen as a radiolucency in the root of a maxillary central incisor.

foration has not occurred, endodontic therapy is indicated. If the tooth is weakened by the resorption, extraction is recommended.

Radiographic Features. Internal resorption is usually detected during radiographic examination. The lesion appears as a round or ovoid radiolucency in the midcrown or midroot portion of a tooth (Figs. 8–17 and 8–18). The outline may appear smooth and well-defined or slightly scalloped. In some instances, the resorptive process may be so extensive that the entire crown or width of the root may be involved.

RADIOGRAPHIC FEATURES OF PULPAL LESIONS

In many dental procedures, information concerning the size and location of the pulp cavity must be obtained before treatment. In cases of very large pulp cavities, there is an increased risk of exposure during restorative treatment. In

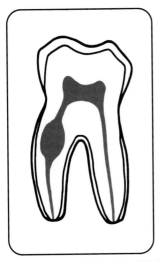

FIGURE 8–16. Internal resorption. (Modified from Eversole LR: Clinical Outline of Oral Pathology: Diagnosis and Treatment, 2d ed. Philadelphia: Lea and Febiger, 1984.)

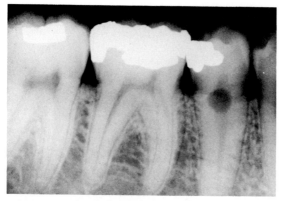

FIGURE 8–18. Internal resorption seen as a round radiolucency in the cervical region of a mandibular second premolar.

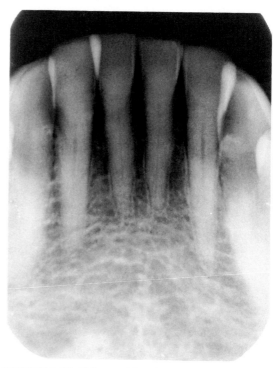

FIGURE 8–20. Thin atrophic pulp chambers seen in mandibular incisors.

cases of pulp cavities reduced in size, endodontic therapy may be difficult. Radiographs allow the dental professional to examine and obtain information concerning the pulp cavity. Without radiographs, examination of the pulp chamber and canals is impossible. Pulpal sclerosis, obliteration of the pulp cavity and pulp stones are common conditions of the pulp cavity that can be viewed on dental radiographs.

Calcification of the Pulp Cavity

Pulpal sclerosis is a diffuse calcification of the pulp chamber and pulp canals of teeth that results in a pulp cavity of decreased size (Fig. 8–19). For unknown reasons, pulpal sclerosis is seen in association with aging. This decrease in size does not appear to be associated with inflammation, trauma or systemic disease.

Clinical Features. No clinical features are associated with pulpal sclerosis. Pulpal sclerosis is generally viewed as an incidental radiographic finding of little clinical significance, unless endodontic therapy is indicated.

Radiographic Features. Diffuse pulpal sclerosis may be viewed as a pulp cavity that is atrophic or reduced in size (Figs. 8–20 and 8–21).

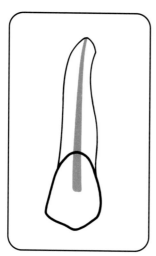

FIGURE 8–19. Pulpal sclerosis.

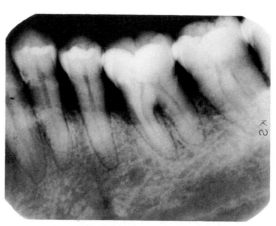

FIGURE 8–21. Pulpal sclerosis.

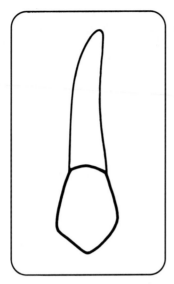

FIGURE 8–22. Pulpal obliteration.

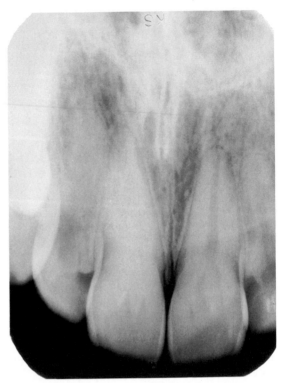

FIGURE 8–23. Pulpal obliteration seen in a maxillary central incisor.

Obliteration of the Pulp Cavity

Some conditions may act as an irritant to the pulp and stimulate the production of secondary dentin and result in the **obliteration of the pulp cavity** (Fig. 8–22). Such conditions include attrition, abrasion, caries, dental restorations, trauma and abnormal mechanical forces.

Clinical Features. Teeth that exhibit obliteration of the pulp cavity are nonvital. No treatment is recommended for a tooth with an obliterated pulp cavity.

Radiographic Features. An obliterated pulp cavity is usually regarded as an incidental radiographic finding. A tooth with an obliterated pulp cavity does not appear to have a pulp chamber or pulp canals when viewed on a radiograph (Figs. 8–23 and 8–24).

Pulp Stones

Pulp stones are calcifications that are found in the pulp chamber or pulp canals of teeth (Fig. 8–25). The incidence of pulp stones is high based on microscopic examination; some studies suggest that 90% of all teeth in individuals age 50 to 70 contain pulp stones. Although most pulp stones are microscopic in size, some may be as large as 2 to 3 mm in diameter. The cause of pulp stones is unknown, and they may be composed of dentin (sometimes referred to as denticles) or foci of dystrophic calcifications. Pulp stones may be attached to the walls of the

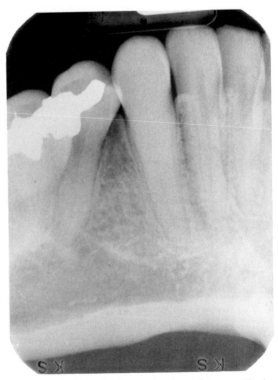

FIGURE 8–24. Pulpal obliteration seen in a mandibular canine.

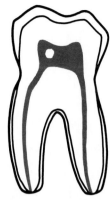

FIGURE 8–25. A pulp stone. (Modified from Eversole LR: Clinical Outline of Oral Pathology: Diagnosis and Treatment, 2d ed. Philadelphia: Lea and Febiger, 1984.)

pulp cavity or completely surrounded by pulpal tissue.

Clinical Features. Pulp stones cannot be identified clinically and are of little significance unless endodontic therapy is indicated. Pulp stones do not cause symptoms and do not require treatment.

Radiographic Features. Some pulp stones are not large enough to be viewed on radiographs. Those that are visible appear as round, ovoid or cylindrical radiopacities; some pulp stones may conform to the shape of the pulp chamber or canal (Figs. 8–26 and 8–27). Pulp stones may be sharply defined or exhibit a diffuse outline. Sizes vary. Pulp stones may occur in singles or multiples and may affect one or more teeth.

RADIOGRAPHIC FEATURES OF PERIAPICAL LESIONS

The use of dental radiographs is particularly important in the identification of periapical problems. Periapical lesions cannot be evaluated on a clinical basis alone. Changes seen in the periapical regions of teeth may be the result of periodontal or pulpal problems. A periapical lesion may appear as either a radiolucency or a radiopacity. Most periapical lesions appear radiolucent and are the result of pulpal inflammation and necrosis, which causes the destruction of bone at the root apex. Periapical radiolucencies, such as the periapical granuloma, periapical cyst and periapical abscess, cannot be diagnosed from a radiograph alone.

When interpreting dental radiographs, it is important to remember that the appearance of radiolucent periapical lesions cannot be used to distinguish between forms of periapical disease. A histologic examination of periapical tissue is necessary to make a diagnosis. A periapical radiolucency viewed on a dental radiograph should not be referred to as a periapical granuloma, periapical cyst or periapical abscess. Instead, the dental professional can describe what is seen on the radiograph as a periapical radiolucency or apical periodontitis.

Periapical Radiolucencies

The periapical granuloma, periapical cyst and periapical abscess are common periapical radiolucencies. These lesions cannot be diagnosed based on their radiographic appearance alone. Each of these lesions has a characteristic histologic appearance and clinical signs and symptoms that vary.

Periapical Granuloma

The **periapical granuloma** can be described as a localized mass of chronically inflamed granulation tissue found at the apex of a nonvital tooth. The periapical granuloma is the result of pulpal

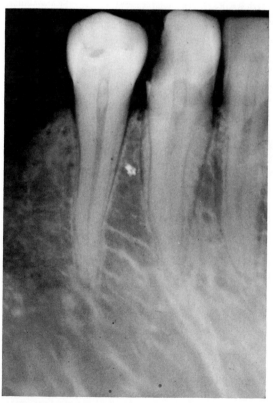

FIGURE 8–26. Cylindrical pulp stones seen in the mandibular canine and premolar.

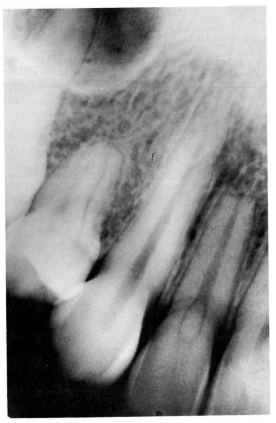

FIGURE 8–27. An ovoid pulp stone seen in a maxillary lateral incisor.

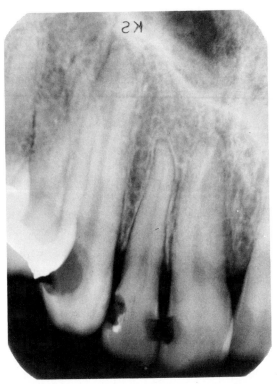

FIGURE 8–28. A widened periodontal ligament space seen at the apex of a maxillary lateral incisor.

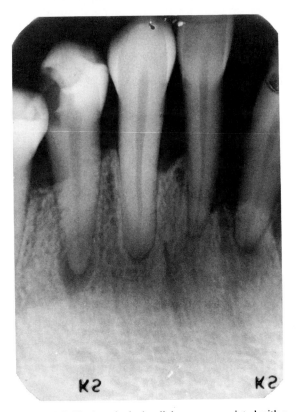

FIGURE 8–29. A periapical radiolucency associated with a mandibular premolar. (Note the lamina dura is not visible.)

death and necrosis and is the most common sequela of pulpitis. The periapical granuloma may give rise to a periapical cyst or periapical abscess.

Clinical Features. A tooth with a periapical granuloma is typically asymptomatic, and the patient usually has a previous history of prolonged sensitivity to heat or cold. In some instances, the tooth may be sensitive to percussion. Treatment for the periapical granuloma may include endodontic therapy or removal of the tooth along with curettage of the apical region.

Radiographic Features. A periapical granuloma is initially seen as a widened periodontal ligament space at the root apex (Fig. 8–28). With time, the widened periodontal ligament space enlarges and appears as a periapical round or ovoid unilocular radiolucency (Fig. 8–29). The lamina dura is not visible between the root apex and the apical lesion.

The periapical granuloma cannot be diagnosed based on its radiographic appearance alone. Histologic examination of periapical tissue is needed in order to make a definitive diagnosis.

Periapical Cyst

The **periapical cyst** is a lesion that develops over a prolonged period of time; cystic degeneration takes place within a periapical granuloma and results in a periapical cyst. The periapical cyst can be identified as an epithelial-lined cavity or sac located at the apex of a nonvital tooth. The periapical cyst, also known as the radicular cyst or apical periodontal cyst, comprises 50% to 70% of all cysts seen in the oral region, making this the most common of all tooth-related cysts. The periapical cyst, like the periapical granuloma, is seen as a result of pulpal death and necrosis.

Clinical Features. Most periapical cysts are asymptomatic and present no clinical signs or symptoms. The affected tooth is seldom painful and is usually discovered during routine radiographic examination. The periapical cyst is always associated with a nonvital pulp. Treatment for the periapical cyst includes endodontic therapy or removal of the tooth along with curettage of the apical region.

Radiographic Features. The typical periapical cyst appears as a round or ovoid unilocular radiolucency (Figs. 8–30 and 8–31). The size may range from less than 5 mm to more than 1 cm. The borders of the periapical cyst may

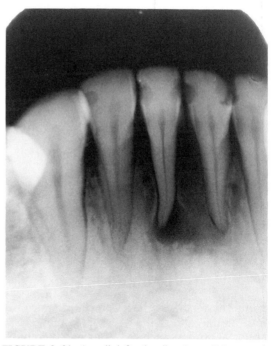

FIGURE 8–31. A well-defined unilocular radiolucency in the periapical location.

appear either corticated or noncorticated. Root resorption may be seen in association with a periapical cyst. Remember that the periapical cyst cannot be diagnosed from a radiograph alone. Histologic examination of periapical tissue is needed in order to make a definitive diagnosis.

Periapical Abscess

The **periapical abscess** is a localized collection of pus seen in the periapical region of a tooth as the result of pulpal death. The periapical abscess may be acute or chronic. The acute periapical abscess exhibits features of an acute suppurative (pus-producing) process and inflammation. The acute abscess may result following an acute inflammation of the pulp or in an area of chronic infection, such as the periapical granuloma. The chronic periapical abscess exhibits features of a long-standing, low-grade suppurative process. A chronic abscess may develop from an acute abscess or periapical granuloma.

Clinical Features. Because of the pus production, the acute periapical abscess is painful—the pain may be intense, throbbing and constant. The tooth is nonvital and sensitive to pressure, percussion and heat. The chronic periapical abscess is usually asymptomatic as a result of pus drainage through bone or the periodontal ligament space. Clinically, a gumboil, or

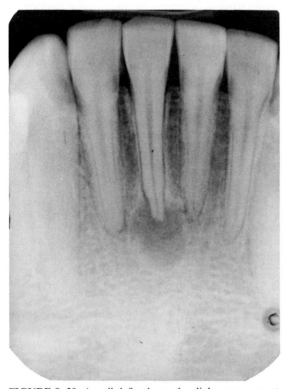

FIGURE 8–30. A well-defined round radiolucency seen at the apex of a mandibular central incisor.

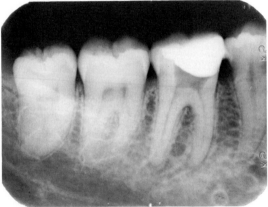

FIGURE 8–32. An increased widening of the periodontal ligament space is noted in the periapical region of the mandibular first molar.

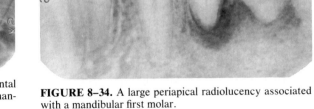

FIGURE 8–34. A large periapical radiolucency associated with a mandibular first molar.

parulis, may be seen in the apical region of a tooth at the site of drainage. Treatment of a periapical abscess includes drainage and endodontic therapy or extraction.

Radiographic Features. With an acute abscess, no periapical radiographic change may be evident. Early radiographic changes include an increased widening of the periodontal ligament space (Fig. 8–32). The typical chronic periapical abscess appears as an apical round or ovoid unilocular radiolucency with diffuse or poorly defined margins (Figs. 8–33 and 8–34). The lamina dura cannot be seen between the root apex and the radiolucent lesion.

As with the periapical granuloma and periapical cyst, the periapical abscess cannot be diagnosed based on its radiographic appearance alone. Histologic examination of periapical tissue is needed in order to make a definitive diagnosis.

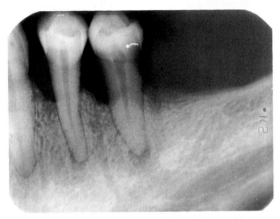

FIGURE 8–33. Periapical radiolucencies associated with the mandibular premolars.

Periapical Radiopacities

Condensing osteitis, sclerotic bone and hypercementosis are a few of the common periapical radiopacities that can be viewed on a dental radiograph. Such localized radiopacities are often encountered during routine dental radiographic examinations. Unlike the periapical radiolucencies, the periapical radiopacities can be diagnosed based on their radiographic appearance, clinical information and patient history.

Condensing Osteitis

Condensing osteitis, also known as chronic focal sclerosing osteomyelitis, is a well-circumscribed focal opacity seen below the apex of a nonvital tooth with a history of a long-standing pulpitis (Fig. 8–35). The opacity represents a proliferation of periapical bone seen as a result of low-grade inflammation or mild irritation. The inflammation that stimulates condensing osteitis is seen in response to pulpal necrosis.

Clinical Features. Condensing osteitis is the most common periapical radiopacity observed in adults. Teeth in the mandible are affected more frequently than the maxilla; the tooth most frequently involved is the mandibular first molar (Fig. 8–36). Teeth associated with condensing osteitis are nonvital and typically have a large carious lesion or large restoration apparent. Because condensing osteitis is believed to represent a physiologic reaction of bone to inflammation, no treatment is indicated.

Radiographic Features. Condensing osteitis appears as a well-demarcated focal opacity located below the root apices on a dental radio-

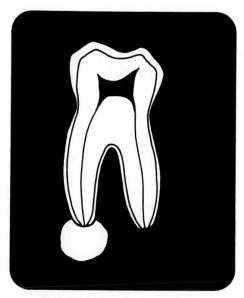

FIGURE 8–35. Condensing osteitis.

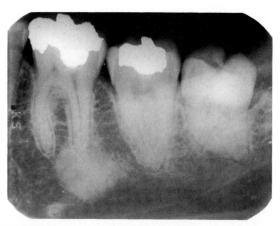

FIGURE 8–37. A well-defined radiopacity is seen in the periapical region of a mandibular first molar.

graph (Fig. 8–37). Condensing osteitis is usually discovered during routine radiographic examination and may vary in size and shape. Condensing osteitis does not appear to be attached to the tooth root.

Sclerotic Bone

Sclerotic bone, also known as osteosclerosis or idiopathic periapical osteosclerosis, is a well-defined focal radiopacity seen below the apices of vital noncarious teeth (Fig. 8–38). The cause of sclerotic bone is unknown; however, it is not believed to be associated with inflammation.

Clinical Features. Sclerotic bone is asymptomatic and is usually discovered during routine radiographic examination.

Radiographic Features. Sclerotic bone appears as a well-defined focal opacity on a dental radiograph (Fig. 8–39). The lesion is not attached to a tooth and may vary in size and shape. The margins may appear smooth or irregular and diffuse. The borders are continuous with adjacent normal bone and no radiolucent outline is seen. Sclerotic bone is not associated with a nonvital tooth.

Hypercementosis

Hypercementosis can be described as an excess deposition of cementum on root surfaces. Hypercementosis may be seen as a result of supraeruption, inflammation or trauma, or in asso-

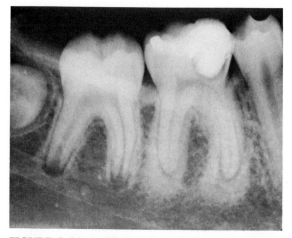

FIGURE 8–36. A diffuse radiopacity is noted along the roots of a mandibular first molar.

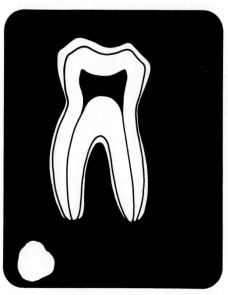

FIGURE 8–38. Sclerotic bone.

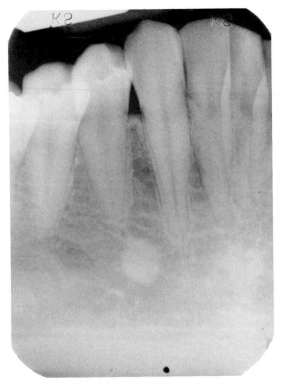

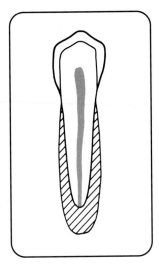

FIGURE 8–40. Hypercementosis. (Modified from Eversole LR: Clinical Outline of Oral Pathology: Diagnosis and Treatment, 2d ed. Philadelphia: Lea and Febiger, 1984.)

FIGURE 8–39. A well-defined radiopacity is seen below the apex of a mandibular premolar.

ciation with Paget's disease. Some cases of hypercementosis have no obvious cause.

Clinical Features. No signs or symptoms are associated with hypercementosis. Most cases are discovered during routine radiographic examination. Hypercementosis may occur in a localized or generalized area; one or more teeth may be affected. Teeth affected by hypercementosis are vital and do not require treatment. Extractions, however, of teeth affected by hypercementosis may be difficult.

Radiographic Features. On a dental radiograph, hypercementosis is seen as an excess amount of cementum along all or part of a root surface (Fig. 8–40). The apical area is most often affected. Tooth roots affected by hypercementosis appear enlarged and bulbous (Figs. 8–41 and 8–42). Root areas affected by hypercementosis are separated from periapical bone by a normal-appearing periodontal ligament space; the surrounding lamina dura appears normal as well.

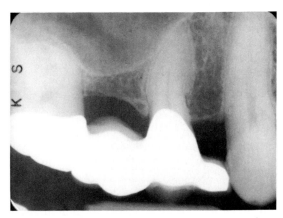

FIGURE 8–41. Hypercementosis is seen as an excess deposition of cementum along the root surfaces of a maxillary premolar.

SUMMARY

Dental radiographs are useful in identifying change. Changes associated with trauma, in-

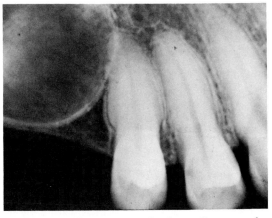

FIGURE 8–42. Hypercementosis of a maxillary premolar.

jury, resorption and lesions that affect the pulpal and periapical tissues can be viewed on dental radiographs. The dental radiograph allows the practitioner to evaluate the roots, pulp cavities and periapical regions of the teeth—all areas that cannot be examined clinically.

The radiographic changes caused by trauma and other injuries are many and varied. Fractures may affect the crowns and roots of teeth or the bones of the maxilla and mandible. Injuries may include partial displacement of teeth into bone and partial or total displacement of teeth out of bone. Radiographic examinations are important in the evaluation of injuries and can be used for diagnostic, treatment and post-treatment purposes.

Dental radiographs are useful in identifying regressive alterations of teeth, such as external and internal resorption as well as pulpal and periapical lesions. Teeth that have undergone the resorption process are usually asymptomatic and are only discovered during radiographic examination. Radiographs allow the dental professional to examine and obtain information about the pulp cavity. Pulpal sclerosis, obliteration of the pulp cavity and pulp stones are common conditions of the pulp cavity that can be viewed on radiographs. Periapical lesions that are not clinically visible can be examined on radiographs. Periapical lesions, such as granulomas, cysts, abscesses, condensing osteitis, sclerotic bone and hypercementosis, can all be identified on radiographs.

The dental professional must be competent in identifying changes associated with trauma, injury, resorption and lesions that affect the pulpal and periapical tissues viewed on dental radiographs. All radiographic findings associated with trauma, injury, resorption or pulpal and periapical lesions should be described in terms of appearance, location and size and be documented in the patient record.

Bibliography

Gibilisco JA: Resorptive processes: *In* Gibilisco JA (ed.): Stafne's Oral Radiographic Diagnosis, pp 125–39. Philadelphia: WB Saunders, 1985.

Gibilisco JA: Condensing osteitis and osteosclerosis. *In* Gibilisco JA (ed.): Stafne's Oral Radiographic Diagnosis, pp 140–46. Philadelphia: WB Saunders, 1985.

Goaz PW and White SC: Trauma to teeth and facial structures. *In* Oral Radiology Principles and Interpretation, 2d ed., pp 719–43. St. Louis: CV Mosby, 1987.

Goaz PW and White SC: Regressive changes of the dentition. *In* Oral Radiology Principles and Interpretation, 2d ed., pp 454–63. St. Louis: CV Mosby, 1987.

Goaz PW and White SC: Infections and inflammation of the jaws and facial bones. *In* Oral Radiology Principles and Interpretation, 2d ed., pp 465–71. St. Louis: CV Mosby, 1987.

Langland OE, Sippy FH and Langlais RP. Radiologic interpretation of dental disease: pulpal and periapical pathology. *In* Textbook of Dental Radiography, 2d ed., pp 452–76. Springfield, IL: Charles C Thomas, 1984.

Manson-Hing LR: Interpretation and value of radiographs. *In* Fundamentals of Dental Radiography, 3d ed., p 207. Philadelphia: Lea and Febiger, 1990.

Miles DA, et al.: Interpretation: normal versus abnormal. *In* Radiographic Imaging for Dental Auxiliaries, pp 187–207. Philadelphia: WB Saunders, 1989.

Miles DA, et al.: Benign fibro-osseous lesions. *In* Oral and Maxillofacial Radiology, pp 125–47. Philadelphia: WB Saunders, 1991.

Miles DA, et al.: Cysts. *In* Oral and Maxillofacial Radiology, pp 21–2. Philadelphia: WB Saunders, 1991.

Miles DA, et al.: Infection/inflammation. *In* Oral and Maxillofacial Radiology, pp 7–8. Philadelphia: WB Saunders, 1991.

Regezi JA and Sciubba JJ: Inflammatory jaw lesions. *In* Oral Pathology: Clinical-Pathologic Correlations, pp 390–94. Philadelphia: WB Saunders, 1989.

Turlingten EG: Injuries to teeth, jaws and zygomas. *In* Gibilisco JA (ed.): Stafne's Oral Radiographic Diagnosis, pp 341–65. Philadelphia: WB Saunders, 1985.

QUIZ QUESTIONS

Matching

For questions 1 to 6, match the terms on the left with the appropriate definition.

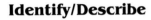 **1.** Trauma   a. Abnormal displacement of teeth

_____ **2.** Fracture   b. An injury produced by an external force

_____ **3.** Luxation   c. Complete displacement of a tooth from alveolar bone

_____ **4.** Intrusion   d. Abnormal displacement of teeth out of bone

_____ **5.** Extrusion   e. The breaking of a part

_____ **6.** Avulsion   f. Abnormal displacement of teeth into bone

Identify/Describe

For questions 7 and 8, circle the correct answer.

7. *Internal resorption / External resorption* may be stimulated by trauma, pulp capping, and/or pulp polyps.

8. *Internal resorption / External resorption* is often associated with reimplanted teeth, abnormal mecahnical forces, trauma, chronic inflammation, tumors, cyts or impacted teeth.

For questions 9 to 11, identify the teeth in the drawings as being displaced by *intrusion, extrusion* or *avulsion*.

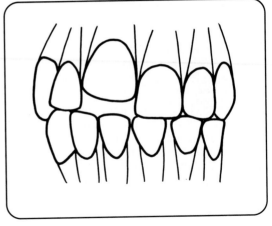

10.

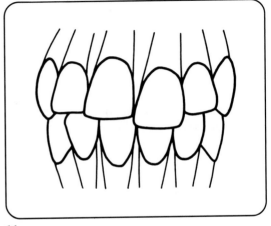

11.

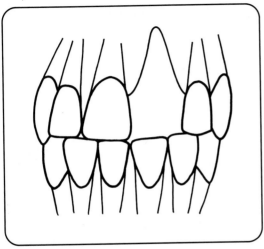

9.

For questions 12 to 14, identify the size of the pulp chambers in the radiographs as being *normal, atrophic* or *enlarged.*

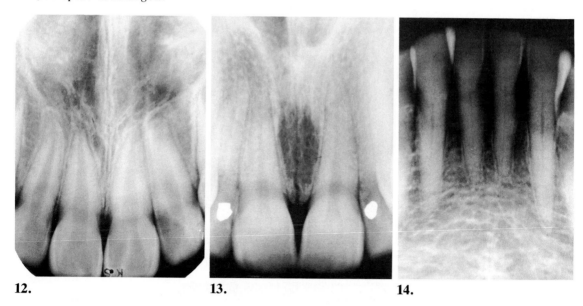

12.   13.   14.

"What Can This Be?"

For questions 15 to 20, identify and/or describe each of the periapical and pulpal lesions.

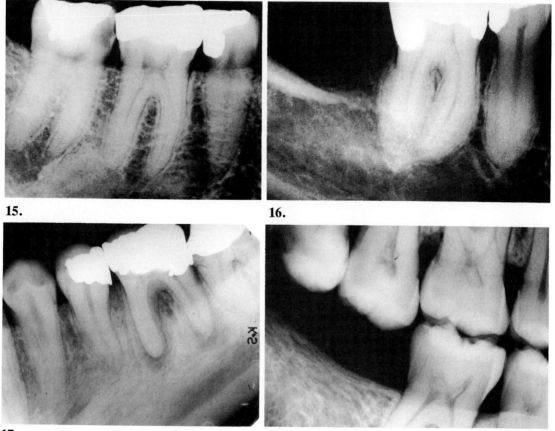

15.   16.

17.   18.

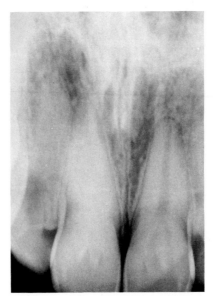

19.

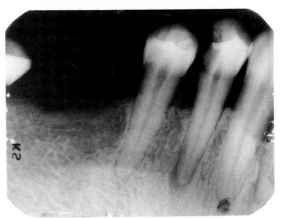

20.

CHAPTER NINE

Film Exposure, Processing and Technique Errors

Objectives

After completion of this chapter, the student will be able to:

▶ List, identify and describe the appearance of the following film exposure errors: unexposed film, film exposed to light, underexposed film and overexposed film.

▶ List, identify and describe the appearance of each of the film processing errors discussed in this chapter.

▶ Describe and identify proper film placement for periapical radiographs.

▶ Define the difference between horizontal and vertical angulation.

▶ Identify technique errors in periapical film placement.

▶ Identify technique errors in vertical and horizontal angulation.

▶ Describe and identify proper film placement for bite-wing radiographs.

▶ Identify technique errors in bite-wing film placement.

▶ Describe and identify the following technique errors and artifacts: film bending, film creasing, phalangioma, cone-cut, double exposure, movement and reversed film.

Key Words

Air bubbles	Light leak
Cone-cut	Overdeveloped film
Developer cut-off	Overexposed film
Developer spots	Overlapped interproximal contacts
Elongation	Phalangioma
Fingernail artifact	Reticulation of emulsion
Fingerprint artifact	Scratched film
Fixer cut-off	Static
Fixer spots	Underdeveloped film
Fogged film	Underexposed film
Foreshortening	Unexposed film
Herringbone pattern	Vertical angulation
Horizontal angulation	Yellow-brown stains

The dental professional must remember that radiographs are taken to benefit the patient. It is important to note that only *diagnostic* radiographs benefit the patient. A diagnostic dental radiograph is one that has been properly placed, exposed and processed; errors in any one of these three areas may result in nondiagnostic films. Since nondiagnostic films, in many cases, must be retaken, any retake results in additional exposure of ionizing radiation, which does not benefit the patient.

In order to avoid films that must be retaken, the dental professional must avoid errors in film exposure, processing and technique. The dental professional must be able to recognize the cause and appearance of film exposure, processing and technique errors and know how to correct such errors. The purpose of this chapter is to review the appearance, cause and correction of common film exposure, positioning and processing errors.

FILM EXPOSURE ERRORS

Film exposure errors result in nondiagnostic films. Exposure problems include films that are not exposed, accidentally exposed to light, overexposed or underexposed. All of these errors produce films that are too light or too dark. The dental professional must be able to recognize film exposure errors, identify their causes and know what steps are necessary to correct such problems.

Exposure Problems

Unexposed Film

Appearance: The film appears clear (Fig. 9–1).
  Cause: The film was not exposed because the x-ray machine was not turned on. Alternate causes include electrical failure or malfunction of the x-ray machine.
  Correction: To insure proper exposure of the film, make certain the x-ray machine is turned on and listen for the audible exposure signal.

Film Exposed to Light

Appearance: The film appears black (Fig. 9–2).
  Cause: The film was accidentally exposed to white light.
  Correction: To protect film, do not unwrap film in a room with white light. Check the darkroom for possible light leaks. Turn off all lights in the darkroom (except for safelights) before unwrapping the film.

FIGURE 9–1. An unexposed film appears clear.

Time and Exposure Factor Problems

Overexposed Film

Appearance: The film appears dark (Fig. 9–3).
  Cause: Overexposed films result from excessive exposure time, kilovoltage, milliamperage or a combination of these factors.
  Correction: To prevent overexposure, check the exposure time, kilovoltage and milliamperage settings on the x-ray machine before exposing radiographs. Reduce exposure time, kilovoltage or milliamperage as needed.

Underexposed Film

Appearance: The film appears light (Fig. 9–4).
  Cause: Underexposed films result from insufficient exposure time, kilovoltage, milliamperage or a combination of these factors.
  Correction: To prevent underexposed films check the exposure time, kilovoltage and milliamperage settings on the x-ray machine before exposing radiographs. Increase exposure time, kilovoltage or milliamperage as needed.

FILM PROCESSING ERRORS

A major cause of faulty radiographs can be traced to problems in processing technique, which may result in nondiagnostic films. Processing errors may occur for a number of reasons, including failure to follow suggested

FIGURE 9–2. A film exposed to light appears black.

time and temperature guidelines, inadequate darkroom facilities, improper care of tanks and processing solutions, chemical contamination and faulty film handling.

Processing errors may cause the partial or total absence of images or obscure images that are present. Films that appear light, dark, yellow-brown or fogged are the result of processing errors. Films that appear scratched or contaminated with dirt, saliva or fingerprints are the result of faulty film handling during processing. Reticulation, fingernail and static artifacts may also be produced as a result of poor processing and film handling techniques.

Many processing errors may be attributed to one or more causes. The dental professional must be able to recognize the appearance of common processing errors, identify potential causes for such errors and know what steps are necessary to correct such problems.

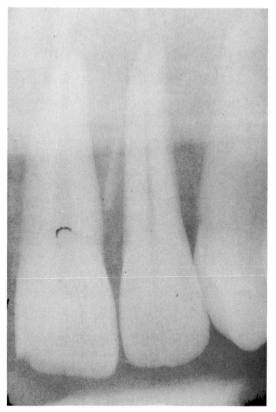

FIGURE 9–4. An underexposed film appears light.

Time and Temperature Problems

Underdeveloped Film

Appearance: The film appears light (Fig. 9–5).

Causes: Underdeveloped films may result from inadequate development time, inaccurate timer, cool developer temperature, inaccurate thermometer or developer solution that is depleted or contaminated.

Correction: To prevent underdeveloped films, check the temperature of the developer as well as the time needed in the developer solution; increase time in developer as needed. Replace faulty and inaccurate thermometers and timers. If developer is depleted or contaminated, replace with fresh developer solution.

Overdeveloped Film

Appearance: The film appears dark (Fig. 9–6).

Cause: Overdeveloped films may result from excess development time, inaccurate timer, hot developer temperature, inaccurate thermometer or developer solution that is concentrated (overactive).

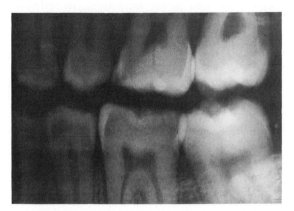

FIGURE 9–3. An overexposed film appears dark.

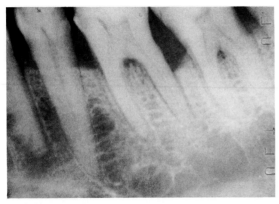

FIGURE 9–5. An underdeveloped film appears light.

Correction: To prevent overdeveloped films, check the temperature of the developer and the time needed in the developer solution; decrease time in the developer as needed. Replace faulty and inaccurate thermometers and timers. If developer is overactive, replace with fresh developer solution.

Reticulation of Emulsion

Appearance: The film appears cracked (Fig. 9–7).

Cause: Reticulation of emulsion results when a film is subjected to a sudden temperature change between the developer solution and the water bath.

Correction: To prevent the reticulation of emulsion, check the temperature of the processing solutions and water bath. Avoid drastic temperature differences between the developer and the water bath.

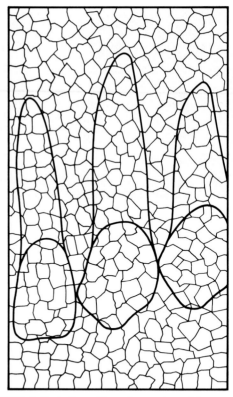

FIGURE 9–7. A film with a damaged emulsion appears cracked.

Chemical Contamination Problems

Developer Spots

Appearance: Dark spots appear on film (Fig. 9–8).

Cause: Developer spots are seen when the developer solution comes in contact with the film *before* processing.

Correction: To avoid developer spots, use a clean work area in the darkroom. In order to ensure a clean working surface, place a paper towel on the work area before unwrapping films.

Fixer Spots

Appearance: White spots appear on film (Fig. 9–9).

Cause: Fixer spots are the result of fixer solution coming in contact with the film *before* processing.

Correction: To avoid fixer spots, use a clean work area in the darkroom. To ensure a clean working surface, place a paper towel on the work area before unwrapping films.

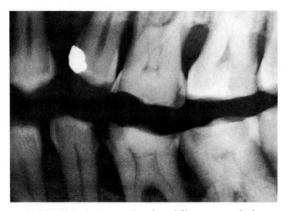

FIGURE 9–6. An overdeveloped film appears dark.

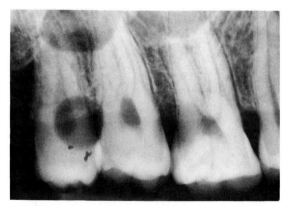

FIGURE 9–8. Developer spots appear dark or black.

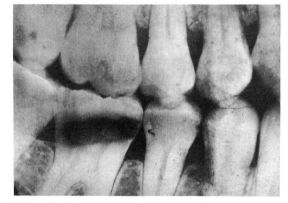

FIGURE 9–10. A number of processing errors may result in a yellow-brown film.

Yellow-Brown Stains

Appearance: The film appears yellowish-brown (Fig. 9–10).

Cause: Yellow-brown films result from the use of exhausted developer or fixer, insufficient fixation time or insufficient rinsing.

Correction: To prevent yellow-brown films, replace depleted developer and fixer solutions with fresh chemicals. Make certain that films have adequate fixation time and adequate rinse time. Processed films should be rinsed for a minimum of 20 minutes in circulating cool water.

Film Handling Problems

Developer Cut-Off

Appearance: A straight white border appears on film (Fig. 9–11).

Cause: Developer cut-off results from a low level of developer solution and represents an undeveloped portion of the film. If the developer

solution is low, the films clipped at the very top of the film rack may not be completely immersed in the developer solution.

Correction: To avoid developer cut-off, check the developer level before processing films.

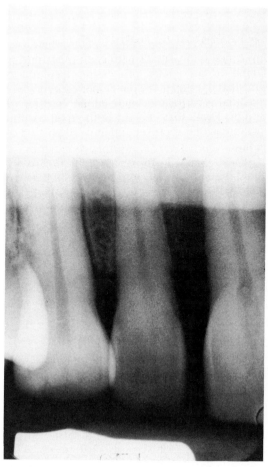

FIGURE 9–11. Developer cut-off appears as a straight white border on a film.

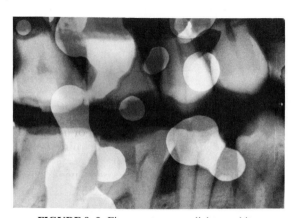

FIGURE 9–9. Fixer spots appear light or white.

Add proper replenisher solution if necessary. Make certain that all films on the film rack are completely immersed in the developer solution.

Fixer Cut-Off

Appearance: A straight, black border appears on film (Fig. 9–12).

Cause: Fixer cut-off results from a low level of fixer solution and represents an unfixed portion of the film. If the fixer solution is low, the films clipped at the very top of the film rack may not be completely immersed in the fixer solution.

Correction: To avoid fixer cut-off, check the fixer level before processing films. Add proper replenisher solution if necessary. Make certain that all films on the film rack are completely immersed in the fixer solution.

Overlapped Films

Appearance: White or dark areas appear on films where overlap has occurred (Figs. 9–13 and 9–14).

Cause: Overlapped films occur when two films come into contact with each other during manual or automatic processing techniques. Films that overlap in the developer exhibit white areas that represent an undeveloped portion of the film. Films that overlap in the fixer exhibit black areas that represent an unfixed portion of the film.

Correction: To avoid overlapped films, care should be taken to ensure that each film is not permitted to come in contact with another film during processing.

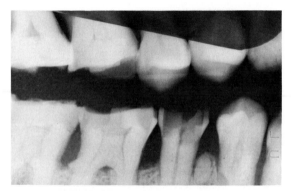

FIGURE 9–13. An overlapped film.

Air Bubbles

Appearance: White spots appear on film (Fig. 9–15).

Cause: Air bubbles are seen when air is trapped on the film surface after the film is placed in the processing solution. Air bubbles prevent the chemicals from affecting the emulsion in that area.

Correction: To avoid air bubbles, gently agitate film racks after placing them in the processing solution.

Fingernail Artifact

Appearance: Black crescent-shaped marks appear on film (Fig. 9–16).

Cause: A fingernail artifact is seen when the film emulsion is damaged by the operator's fingernail during rough handling of the film.

Correction: To prevent a fingernail artifact, gently handle film by the edges only.

Fingerprint Artifact

Appearance: A black fingerprint appears on film (Fig. 9–17).

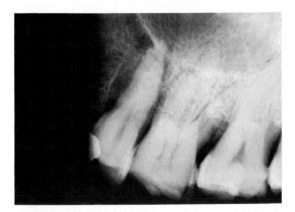

FIGURE 9–12. Fixer cut-off appears as a straight black border on a film.

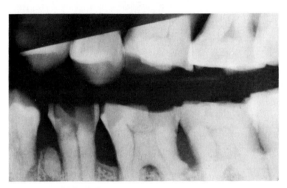

FIGURE 9–14. An overlapped film.

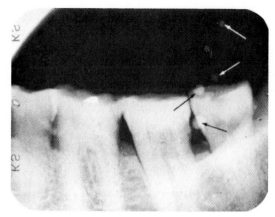

FIGURE 9–15. Air bubbles appear as tiny white spots. (From Langlais RP and Kasle MK: Exercises in Radiographic Interpretation, 2d ed. Philadelphia: WB Saunders, 1985.)

Cause: A fingerprint artifact is seen when the film is touched by fingers contaminated with fluoride or developer.

Correction: To prevent fingerprint artifacts, wash and dry hands thoroughly before processing films. Work in a clean area to avoid contaminating the hands and handle the films by the edges only.

Static

Appearance: Thin black branching lines appear on the film (Fig. 9–18).

Cause: Static electricity may result from opening a film packet quickly. It may also be created in a carpeted office when a film packet is opened before touching a conductive object. Static electricity occurs most frequently during periods of low humidity.

Correction: To prevent static electricity, always open film packets slowly. In a carpeted office, touch a conductive object before unwrapping films.

Scratched Film

Appearance: White lines appear on film (Fig. 9–19).

Cause: A scratch results when the soft film emulsion is removed from the film base by a sharp object, such as a film clip or film hanger.

Correction: To prevent a scratched film, use care when placing a film rack in the processing solutions and avoid contact with other film hangers.

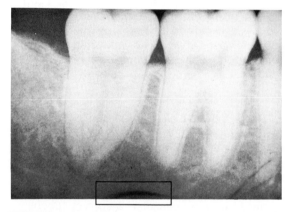

FIGURE 9–16. A fingernail artifact appears as a black crescent-shaped mark.

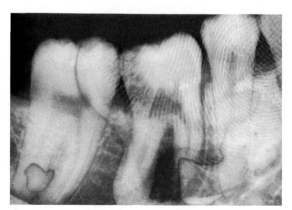

FIGURE 9–17. A fingerprint artifact appears black.

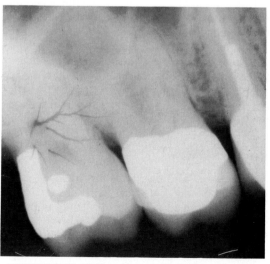

FIGURE 9–18. Static appears as black, branching lines.

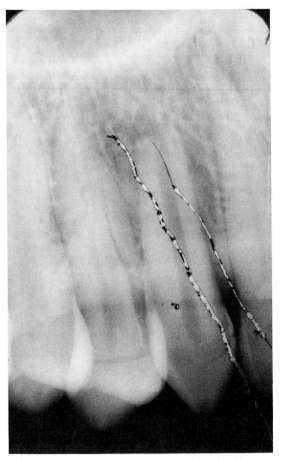

FIGURE 9–19. Scratches appear as thin white lines.

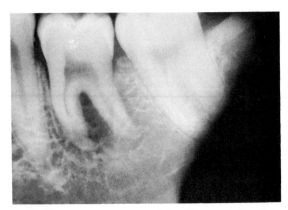

FIGURE 9–20. The portion of the film exposed to light appears black.

Correction: To prevent fogged films, check the filter and bulb wattage of the safelight, minimize film exposure to safelight and check the darkroom for light leaks. Check the expiration date on film packages and store films in a cool, dry and protected area. Avoid contamination of processing solutions by replacing tank covers after each use. Always check developer temperature before processing films.

TECHNIQUE ERRORS

Just as exposure and processing errors may result in nondiagnostic films, errors in technique may also result in films that are nondiagnostic. Technique errors include incorrect positioning of the film or tubehead or incorrect tubehead angulation. Technique errors may involve periapical or bite-wing films.

Light Problems

Light Leak

Appearance: The exposed area appears black (Fig. 9–20).
Cause: A light leak results from the accidental exposure of the film to white light. Torn or defective film packets may allow a portion of the film to be exposed to light.
Correction: To prevent light leaks, examine film packets for minute tears or defects before use. Do not use film packets that are torn or defective. Never unwrap films in the presence of white light.

Fogged Film

Appearance: The film appears gray and lacks image detail and contrast (Fig. 9–21).
Cause: Fogged films result from improper safelighting and light leaks in the darkroom. Film fog may also result from improper film storage, outdated films, contaminated processing solutions or hot developer temperature.

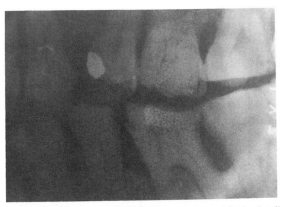

FIGURE 9–21. A fogged film appears gray and lacks detail and contrast.

Periapical Technique Errors

Periapical technique errors may involve film placement or angulation problems. A properly placed periapical radiograph shows the entire tooth, including the apex and surrounding structures (Fig. 9–22). Periapical film placement errors may result in the absence of apical structures or an occlusal plane that appears tipped or tilted. Angulation problems may result in overlapped structures, elongation or foreshortening.

Film Placement Problems

Correct Film Placement. Each periapical radiograph must be positioned to image specific teeth and related anatomic structures. Proper film placement is critical in good periapical technique. The dental professional must be able to properly place periapical films in the incisor, canine, premolar and molar areas of the maxilla

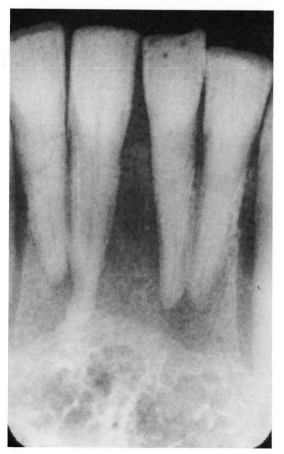

FIGURE 9–22. Proper periapical film placement demonstrates the entire tooth, including the apex and surrounding structures.

and mandible. As a rule, films should be centered over the area of interest (Table 9–1).

Depending on the region of the mouth, periapical films may be placed in either a vertical or horizontal direction. Periapical films used in the anterior regions are placed with the long axis of the film in a vertical direction, and periapical films used in the posterior regions are placed with the long axis of the film in a horizontal direction. The edges of periapical films must be placed parallel with the incisal or occlusal surfaces of the teeth and extend beyond the incisal or occlusal surfaces approximately 3 to 6 mm (⅛″ to ¼″) (Fig. 9–23).

When positioned in the mouth, periapical films must be kept as flat as possible in order to minimize the chance of film bending and distortion. The white side of the film (tube side) must be placed behind the tooth to be exposed. The identification dot (found on the back of the film) should always be positioned at the incisal or occlusal edge of the film (Fig. 9–24). If the identification dot is not positioned at the incisal edge of the film, it may interfere with diagnostic information.

Incorrect Film Placement. Incorrect placement of a periapical film may result in a nondiagnostic film. Periapical film placement errors may result from not only improper positioning of the film over the area of intended interest but inadequate coverage of the apical regions or dropped film corners as well.

Absence of Apical Structures
Appearance: No apices appear on film (Fig. 9–25).

Cause: An absence of apical structures results when a periapical film is not placed high enough on the palate or low enough on the floor of the mouth to adequately cover the apical regions of the teeth. In addition to the absence of apical structures, an excessive margin of film edge (which appears as a radiolucent band) is seen on the resultant radiograph.

Correction: To prevent the absence of apical structures on a periapical radiograph, make certain that no more than 3 to 6 mm of the film edge extends beyond the incisal or occlusal surfaces of the teeth. Such film placement insures adequate coverage of the tooth apices.

Dropped Film Corner
Appearance: Occlusal plane appears tipped or tilted (Fig. 9–26).

Cause: A dropped film corner results when the edge of a periapical film is not placed parallel to the incisal or occlusal surfaces of the teeth. If the patient is not instructed to firmly hold the

TABLE 9–1. Periapical Film Placement

	Bisection-of-the-Angle Technique	Paralleling Technique
Maxillary Arch		
Incisor	Center the film over the midline.	Center the film over the contact between the central and lateral incisors.
Canine	Center the film over the canine.	Center the film over the canine.
Premolar	Center the film over the second premolar.	Center the film over the second premolar.
Molar	Center the film over the second molar.	Center the film over the second molar.
Mandibular Arch		
Incisor	Center the film over the midline.	Center the film over the midline.
Canine	Center the film over the canine.	Center the film over the canine.
Premolar	Center the film over the second premolar.	Center the film over the second premolar.
Molar	Center the film over the second molar.	Center the film over the second molar.

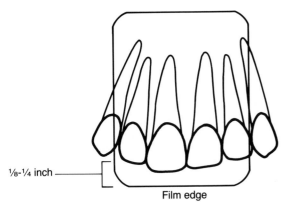

⅛-¼ inch ⎯⎯⎯

Film edge

FIGURE 9–23. A periapical film should extend ⅛″ to ¼″ beyond the incisal or occlusal surfaces of the teeth. (Modified from Manson-Hing LR: Fundamentals of Dental Radiography, 3d ed. Philadelphia: Lea and Febiger, 1990.)

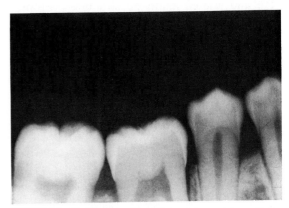

FIGURE 9–25. Improper film placement: no apices appear on this film.

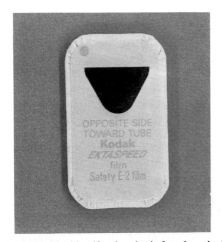

FIGURE 9–24. The identification dot is found on the back side of the film. (From Miles DA et al.: Radiographic Imaging for Dental Auxiliaries, 1st ed. Philadelphia: WB Saunders, 1989.)

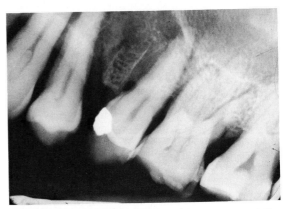

FIGURE 9–26. Improper film placement: a dropped film corner is seen when the edge of the film is not placed parallel to the incisal or occlusal surfaces of the teeth.

periapical film in place against the crown of the tooth, a corner of the film may drop or slip.

Correction: To prevent a dropped film corner, make certain that the edge of the film is placed parallel to the incisal or occlusal surfaces of the teeth. Instruct the patient to firmly hold the film in place.

Angulation Problems

Angulation is a term that is used to describe the alignment of the central beam in the horizontal and vertical planes. Angulation can be varied by rotating the tubehead or position indicating device (PID) in either a horizontal or vertical direction.

Correct Horizontal Angulation. Horizontal angulation refers to the positioning of the tubehead and direction of the central ray in a horizontal (side-to-side) plane (Fig. 9–27). With correct horizontal angulation, the central ray is directed perpendicular to the curvature of the arch and *through* the contact areas of the teeth (Fig. 9–28). With proper horizontal angulation, the contact areas on the resultant film appear "opened"; incorrect horizontal angulation results in overlapped contact areas (Fig. 9–29). A film with overlapped interproximal contact areas cannot be used to examine the interproximal areas of the teeth and is considered nondiagnostic.

Incorrect Horizontal Angulation

Appearance: Overlapped contacts appear on film (Fig. 9–30).

Cause: Overlapped interproximal contacts result from incorrect horizontal angulation. If the central ray is not directed through the interproximal spaces, the proximal surfaces of adjacent teeth appear overlapped on the resultant periapical film. Overlapped contacts prevent the examination of interproximal regions.

Correction: In order to avoid overlapped contacts on periapical films, direct the x-ray beam *through* the interproximal spaces. The use of the paralleling technique minimizes errors in horizontal angulation.

Correct Vertical Angulation. Vertical angulation refers to the positioning of the tubehead and direction of the central ray in a vertical (up and down) plane (Fig. 9–31). The film position and vertical angulation differ depending on the radiographic technique used. With the paralleling technique, the vertical angulation of the central beam is directed perpendicular to the film. With the bisection-of-the-angle technique, the vertical angulation is determined by the bisection of an imaginary angle

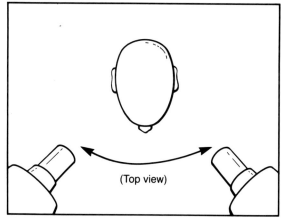

FIGURE 9–27. Horizontal angulation of the cone refers to cone placement in a side-to-side (ear-to-ear) direction.

formed by the long axis of the tooth and the plane of the film. Incorrect vertical angulation results in elongated or foreshortened images; images that are elongated or foreshortened are nondiagnostic.

Foreshortened Images

Appearance: Short teeth with blunted roots appear on the film (Fig. 9–32).

Cause: Foreshortened images result from *excessive* vertical angulation. The teeth appear short with blunted roots. The film is considered nondiagnostic because the image is *not* representative of the true length of the tooth.

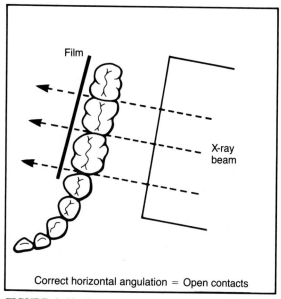

Correct horizontal angulation = Open contacts

FIGURE 9–28. Correct horizontal angulation. (Modified from Manson-Hing LR: Fundamentals of Dental Radiography, 3d ed. Philadelphia: Lea and Febiger, 1990.)

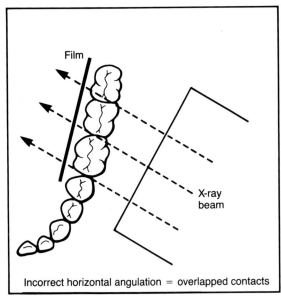

Incorrect horizontal angulation = overlapped contacts

FIGURE 9–29. Incorrect horizontal angulation. (Modified from Manson-Hing LR: Fundamentals of Dental Radiography, 3d ed. Philadelphia: Lea and Febiger, 1990.)

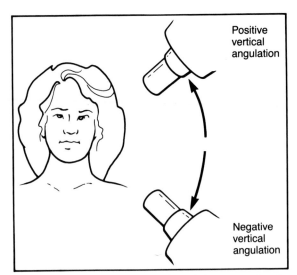

FIGURE 9–31. Vertical angulation of the cone refers to cone placement in an up-and-down (head-to-toe) direction.

paralleling technique minimizes errors in inadequate vertical angulation.

Bite-Wing Technique Errors

Bite-wing technique errors may involve film placement or angulation problems. The bite-wing film must show the crowns of both the maxillary and mandibular teeth and exhibit open interproximal contacts (Fig. 9–34). Bite-wing film placement and angulation errors may result in missing tooth surfaces, a tipped occlusal plane, overlapped interproximal contacts or distorted images.

Film Placement Problems

Correct Film Placement. The bite-wing radiograph is the radiograph of choice for the evaluation of dental caries. In order for a bite-wing radiograph to be considered diagnostic, the film placement must be correct, the occlusal plane must be positioned horizontally along the midline of the long axis of the tooth and the interproximal areas must demonstrate open contacts (Fig. 9–35).

Premolar Bite-Wing. The premolar bite-wing must be positioned so the resultant film shows *both* the maxillary and mandibular premolars and the distal contact area of both canines (Fig. 9–36). In order to ensure that the distal surfaces of the canines are evident on the resultant radiograph, the film must be positioned

Correction: In order to avoid foreshortened images, do not use excessive vertical angulation with the bisection-of-the-angle technique. The use of the paralleling technique minimizes errors in excessive vertical angulation.

Elongated Images

Appearance: Long, distorted teeth appear on the film (Fig. 9–33).

Cause: Elongated images result from *insufficient* vertical angulation. On the resultant radiograph, the teeth appear long and distorted. The film is considered nondiagnostic because the image is *not* representative of the actual length of the tooth.

Correction: In order to avoid elongated images, use adequate vertical angulation with the bisection-of-the-angle technique. The use of the

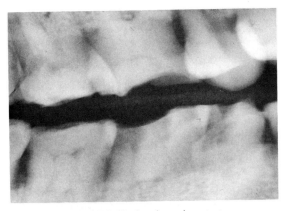

FIGURE 9–30. Overlapped contacts.

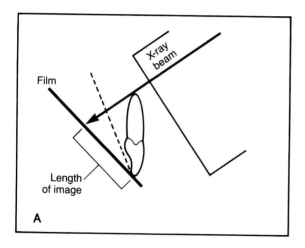

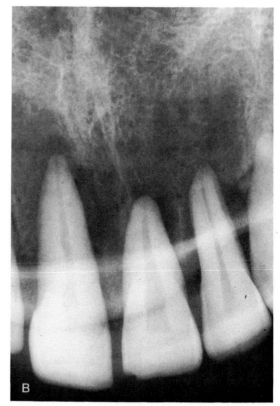

FIGURE 9–32. *A*, If the vertical angulation is too steep, the image of the tooth on the film is shorter than the actual tooth. (Modified from Manson-Hing LR: Fundamentals of Dental Radiography, 3d ed. Philadelphia: Lea and Febiger, 1990.) *B*, Foreshortened images.

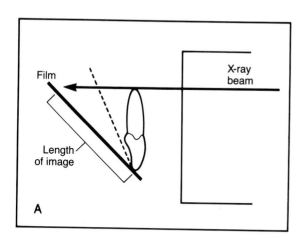

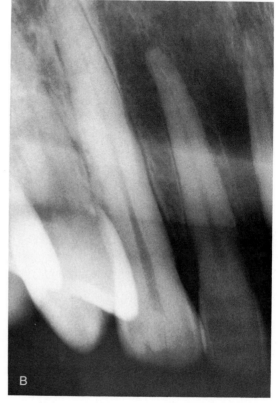

FIGURE 9–33. *A*, If the vertical angulation is too flat, the image of the tooth on the film is longer than the actual tooth. (Modified from Manson-Hing LR: Fundamentals of Dental Radiography, 3d ed. Philadelphia: Lea and Febiger, 1990.) *B*, Elongated images.

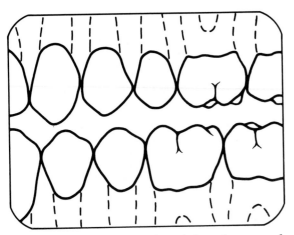

FIGURE 9–34. A bite-wing radiograph shows the crowns of both the maxillary and mandibular teeth. (Modified from Goaz PW and White SC: Oral Radiology: Principles and Interpretation, 2d ed. St. Louis: CV Mosby, 1987.)

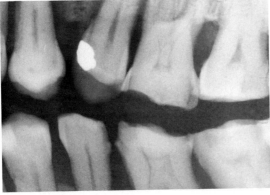

FIGURE 9–35. A diagnostic bite-wing radiograph demonstrates proper film placement and open interproximal contacts.

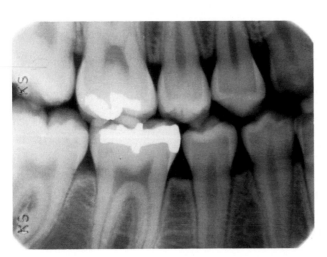

FIGURE 9–36. This film demonstrates correct premolar bite-wing film placement. (From Miles DA et al.: Radiologic Imaging for Dental Auxiliaries, 1st ed. Philadelphia: WB Saunders, 1989.)

so that the anterior edge of the film covers the maxillary and mandibular canines (Fig. 9–37).

Molar Bite-Wing. The molar bite-wing must be positioned so that the resultant film shows *both* the maxillary and mandibular molars (Fig. 9–38). The molar bite-wing must be centered over the *second mandibular molar* so that the third molar region can be examined for possible impacted teeth, supernumerary (extra) teeth, cysts and tumors (Fig. 9–39).

Incorrect Film Placement. Incorrect bite-wing film placement may result in the absence of specific teeth or tooth surfaces on a film and, as a result, render a film nondiagnostic.

Premolar Bite-Wing

Appearance: The distal surfaces of the canines are not visible on the film (Fig. 9–40).

Cause: The distal surfaces of the canines are not visible on the film because the bite-wing was positioned too far posteriorly in the mouth.

Correction: In order to prevent this film placement error, make certain that the anterior edge of the bite-wing film covers the maxillary and mandibular canines.

Molar Bite-Wing

Appearance: The third molar region is not visible on the film (Fig. 9–41).

Cause: The third molar region is not visible on the film because the bite-wing was positioned too far anteriorly in the mouth.

Correction: In order to prevent this film placement error, *always* center the molar bite-wing over the second molar (even when there are no erupted third molars).

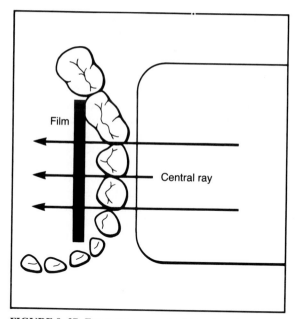

FIGURE 9–37. For correct premolar bite-wing placement, the canine is covered by the anterior edge of the film.

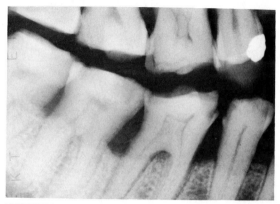

FIGURE 9–39. For correct molar bite-wing film placement, the film is centered over the second molar.

Angulation Problems

In order to produce a diagnostic bite-wing radiograph, the dental professional must be prepared to choose the correct horizontal and vertical angulation. Incorrect horizontal angulation results in overlapped interproximal contacts. Incorrect vertical angulation results in distorted images.

Correct Angulation
Horizontal Angulation. The correct horizontal angulation is chosen based on the curvature of the patient's arch. The central ray is directed through the contact areas of the teeth

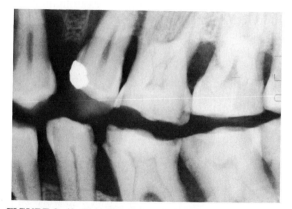

FIGURE 9–40. This film demonstrates incorrect premolar bite-wing film placement; the distal surfaces of the canines are not visible.

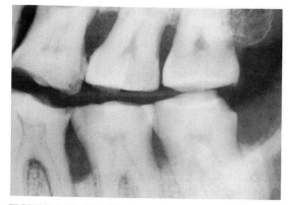

FIGURE 9–38. This film demonstrates correct molar bite-wing film placement.

FIGURE 9–41. This film demonstrates incorrect molar bite-wing film placement; the third molar area is not visible.

(Fig. 9–42). If properly directed, the contact areas on the resultant bite-wing radiograph appear "opened," and a thin radiolucent line is seen between the adjacent tooth surfaces (Fig. 9–43).

Vertical Angulation. With the bite-wing radiograph, a positive 10 degrees (+10) vertical angulation is always used (Fig. 9–44). The +10 vertical angulation is used to compensate for the slight bend of the upper half of the film and the tilt of the maxillary teeth (Fig. 9–45).

Incorrect Horizontal Angulation

Overlapped Contacts

Appearance: Overlapped contacts appear on film (Fig. 9–46).

Cause: Overlapped interproximal contacts result from incorrect horizontal angulation. If the central ray is not directed through the interproximal spaces, the proximal surfaces of adjacent teeth appear overlapped on the bite-wing film. Overlapped contacts prevent the examination of interproximal regions. A bite-wing film with overlapped contacts is nondiagnostic.

Correction: In order to avoid overlapped contacts on bite-wing radiographs, direct the x-ray beam *through* the interproximal spaces. If the contacts are opened, a thin radiolucent line is seen between the proximal surfaces of the teeth.

Incorrect Vertical Angulation
Appearance: Images appear distorted (Fig. 9–47).

Cause: Distorted images result from improper vertical angulation. If a negative vertical angulation is used, the occlusal surfaces of the maxillary teeth are evident and the apical regions of the mandibular teeth are seen. A bite-wing radiograph exposed with an excessive negative vertical angulation is nondiagnostic.

Correction: In order to avoid vertical angulation errors with bite-wing radiographs, always use a positive vertical angulation of *5 to 10 degrees.* This vertical angulation compensates for the slight tilt of the maxillary teeth and the slight lingual bend of the upper half of the film caused by the hard palate.

Miscellaneous Problems

Film Bending

Appearance: Film appears distorted (Fig. 9–48).

Cause: Film bending results from excessive bending of the intraoral film. Films are often bent because of the curvature of the hard palate or alveolar arch or because of strong finger pressure placed on the film. Film bending causes distortion of the radiographic image and often results in a nondiagnostic film.

Correction: In order to avoid film bending, always check film placement before exposure. If the patient's finger pressure is excessive, instruct the patient to gently hold the film in place. Film holding devices may be helpful in preventing film bending.

Film Creasing

Appearance: A thin, radiolucent line appears on the film (Fig. 9–49).

Cause: A film crease results from excessive bending. Excessive bending of a film may cause the film emulsion to crack.

Correction: In order to avoid film creasing, avoid excessive bending or creasing of the film. Instead, gently soften the corners of the film before placing a film in a patient's mouth.

Phalangioma

Appearance: The bones of a patient's finger appear on the film (Fig. 9–50).

Cause: A phalangioma is seen as a result of the patient's finger being placed in front of the film instead of behind the film. The term was coined by Dr. David F. Mitchell of Indiana Uni-

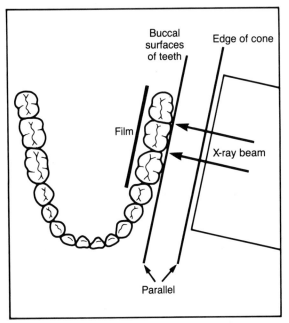

FIGURE 9–42. Correct horizontal angulation. (Modified from Manson-Hing, LR: Fundamentals of Dental Radiography, 3d ed. Philadelphia: Lea and Febiger, 1990.)

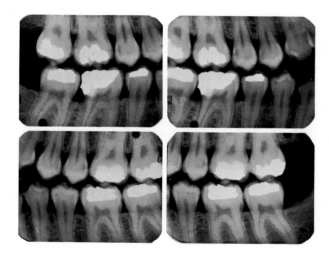

FIGURE 9–43. An open contact appears as a thin, radiolucent line between adjacent tooth surfaces. (From Gibilisco JA (ed.): Stafne's Oral Radiographic Diagnosis, 5th ed. Philadelphia: WB Saunders, 1985.)

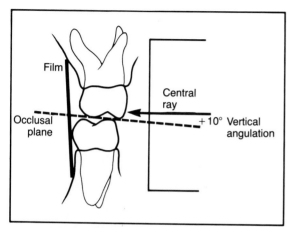

FIGURE 9–44. A +10-degree vertical angulation is recommended for bite-wing radiographs. (Modified from Manson-Hing LR: Fundamentals of Dental Radiography, 3d ed. Philadelphia: Lea and Febiger, 1990.)

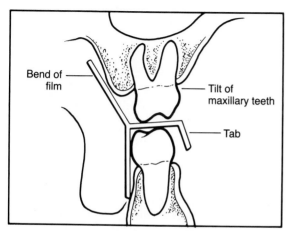

FIGURE 9–45. A positive vertical angulation is used to compensate for the slight bend of the upper portion of the film and the tilt of the maxillary teeth.

versity School of Dentistry and refers to the distal phalanx of the finger seen in the film. (A phalanx [plural, phalanges] is any bone of the finger.)

Correction: In order to avoid a phalangioma, always check to make certain that the patient is holding or stabilizing the film with his or her finger behind the film, not in front of it (Fig. 9–51).

Cone-Cut

Appearance: A curved unexposed area appears on the film (Fig. 9–52).

Cause: A cone-cut is seen when a portion of the film has not been exposed to the x-ray beam (Fig. 9–53). If the beam is misdirected and did not cover the entire film, a curved clear area that resembles the outline of the cone is seen. A cone-cut may obscure important information in the area being examined and render the radiograph nondiagnostic.

Correction: In order to avoid a cone-cut, position the tubehead and PID carefully. The center of the primary beam must be directed at the center of the film to insure that the entire film is exposed. A film holding device with locator ring (e.g., Rinn device) can be used to align the beam and prevent cone-cuts.

Double Exposure

Appearance: A double image appears on the film (Fig. 9–54).

Cause: A double exposure results when a film has been exposed in the patient's mouth twice. A double exposure is a serious technique error and results in *two* retakes, one of each area previously exposed.

Correction: In order to avoid a double expo-

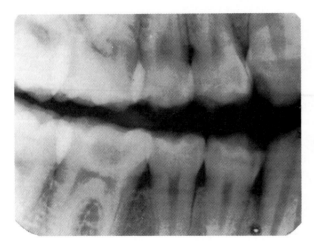

FIGURE 9–46. Overlapped interproximal contacts. (From Miles DA et al.: Radiographic Imaging for Dental Auxiliaries, 1st ed. Philadelphia: WB Saunders, 1989.)

sure, always use a systematic approach for the exposure of radiographs. Once a film has been exposed, place it in a designated area (away from films that have yet to be exposed). Exposed films can be placed in a cup, bag or other suitable receptacle.

Movement

Appearance: A blurred image appears on the film (Fig. 9–55).

Cause: A blurred image results from movement of either the patient or the tubehead. Blurred images are nondiagnostic.

Correction: In order to prevent movement errors, stabilize the patient's head before exposing the radiograph and instruct the patient to remain still. If the tubehead has moved or drifted after you have positioned it, do not expose the radio-

graph. Reposition the tubehead before exposing the film. (Never expose a radiograph if the patient or tubehead has moved.)

Reversed Film

Appearance: Film appears light and exhibits a herringbone or tire-track pattern (Fig. 9–56).

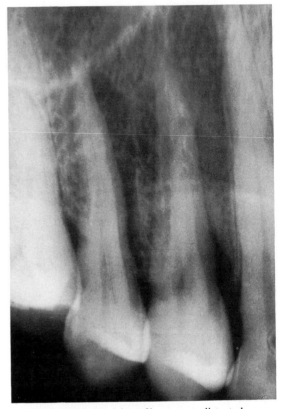

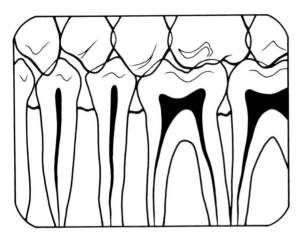

FIGURE 9–47. Negative vertical angulation.

FIGURE 9–48. A bent film appears distorted.

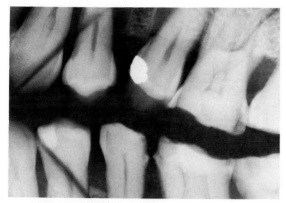

FIGURE 9–49. A film crease appears as a thin radiolucent line.

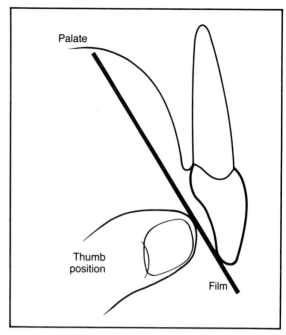

FIGURE 9–51. This diagram demonstrates the correct placement of a patient's finger to stabilize a periapical film. (Modified from Manson-Hing LR: Fundamentals of Dental Radiography, 3d ed. Philadelphia: Lea and Febiger, 1990.)

Cause: A light film with a **herringbone** or tire-track **pattern** results when a reversed film is placed in the mouth. X-rays are attenuated by the lead foil backing in the film packet before exposing the film, and as a result, the film appears light. The herringbone or tire-track pattern on the radiograph is representative of the actual pattern embossed on the lead foil (Fig. 9–57).

Correction: In order to avoid a reversed film, always place the white side of the film adjacent to the teeth to be exposed. Before placing a film in the patient's mouth, always note the front and back sides of the film.

SUMMARY

In order to benefit the patient, dental radiographs must be diagnostic. Film exposure, processing and technique errors often result in nondiagnostic films. The errors associated with film exposure, processing and technique are many and varied. Film exposure problems include films that are unexposed, exposed to light, underexposed and overexposed. Processing errors may result from failure to follow suggested time and temperature guidelines, inadequate

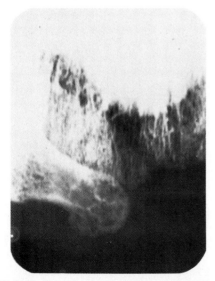

FIGURE 9–50. This film demonstrates a "phalangioma." (From Langlais RP and Kasle MK: Exercises in Radiographic Interpretation, 2d ed. Philadelphia: WB Saunders, 1985.)

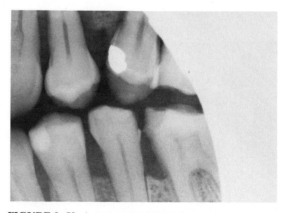

FIGURE 9–52. A cone-cut appears as a curved unexposed (clear) area on a radiograph.

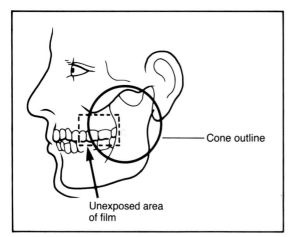

FIGURE 9–53. The cone must be positioned to "cover" the entire film. If not, the unexposed area of the film will appear as a curved clear area. (Modified from Manson-Hing LR: Fundamentals of Dental Radiography, 3d ed. Philadelphia: Lea and Febiger, 1990.)

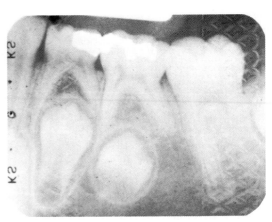

FIGURE 9–56. A reversed film appears light with a herringbone or tire-track pattern. (From Langlais RP and Kasle MK: Exercises in Radiographic Interpretation, 2d ed. Philadelphia: WB Saunders, 1985.)

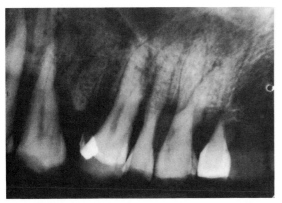

FIGURE 9–54. This film demonstrates a double exposure.

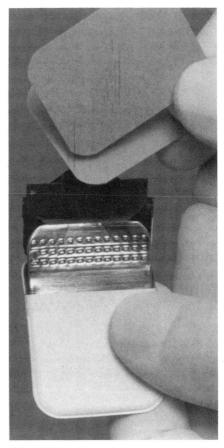

FIGURE 9–57. The embossed tire-track pattern is seen on the lead foil backing found within the film packet. (From Miles DA et al.: Radiographic Imaging for Dental Auxiliaries, 1st ed. Philadelphia: WB Saunders, 1989.)

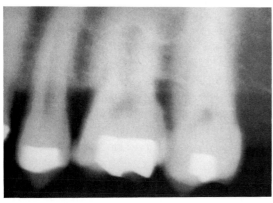

FIGURE 9–55. Movement results in a blurred image.

darkroom facilities, improper care of tanks and processing solutions, chemical contamination or faulty film handling. Technique errors include incorrect positioning of the film or tubehead or incorrect angulation.

Recognition of such common errors is necessary for interpreting radiographs. The dental professional must be competent in identifying errors associated with exposure, processing and technique problems. In addition to recognizing such errors, the dental professional must also be competent in knowing how to correct such errors. This chapter has reviewed the appearance, cause and correction of common film exposure, processing and technique errors.

Bibliography

De Lyre WR and Johnson ON: Dental x-ray film processing. *In* Essentials of Dental Radiography for Dental Assistants and Hygienists, pp 111–45. Norwalk, CT: Appleton and Lange, 1990.

De Lyre WR and Johnson ON: Identifying and correcting faulty radiographs. *In* Essentials of Dental Radiography for Dental Assistants and Hygienists, pp 207–25. Norwalk, CT: Appleton and Lange, 1990.

De Lyre WR: Intraoral radiographic procedures. *In* Essentials of Dental Radiography for Dental Assistants and Hygienists, pp 227–50. Norwalk, CT: Appleton and Lange, 1990.

Gibilisco JA: The processing of x-ray films. *In* Gibilisco JA (ed.): Stafne's Oral Radiographic Diagnosis, pp 463–70. Philadelphia: WB Saunders, 1985.

Goaz PW and White SC: Processing x-ray film. *In* Oral Radiology Principles and Interpretation, 2d ed., pp 121–41. St. Louis: CV Mosby, 1987.

Langland OE, Sippy FH and Langlais RP: Film processing and duplication. *In* Textbook of Dental Radiography, 2d ed., pp 281–321. Springfield, IL: Charles C Thomas, 1984.

Langland OE, Sippy FH and Langlais RP: Analysis of errors and artifacts. *In* Textbook of Dental Radiography, 2d ed., pp 322–51. Springfield, IL: Charles C Thomas, 1984.

Manson-Hing LR: Films, processing, darkroom, and duplicating. *In* Fundamentals of Dental Radiography, 3d ed., pp 16–39. Philadelphia: Lea and Febiger, 1990.

Manson-Hing LR: Radiographic quality and artifacts. *In* Fundamentals of Dental Radiography, 3d ed., pp 40–47. Philadelphia: Lea and Febiger, 1990.

Miles DA et al.: Technique/processing errors and troubleshooting. *In* Radiographic Imaging for Dental Auxiliaries, pp 96–121. Philadelphia: WB Saunders, 1989.

QUIZ QUESTIONS

"What Can This Be?"

For questions 1 to 5, identify the film exposure, processing or technique error.

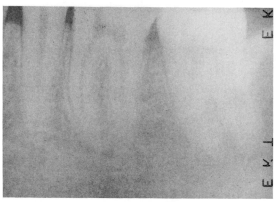

1.

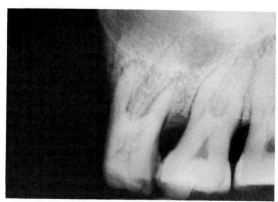

2.

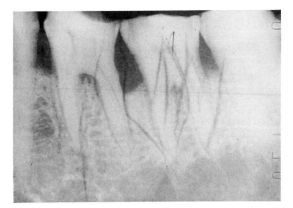

3.

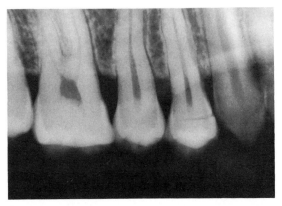

4.

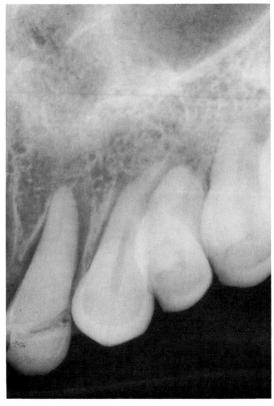

5.

Matching

For questions 6 to 12, describe the appearance of film error using one of these words:

_____ **6.** Fogged film
_____ **7.** Overdeveloped film
_____ **8.** Underdeveloped film
_____ **9.** Film exposed to light
_____ **10.** Unexposed film
_____ **11.** Underexposed film
_____ **12.** Overexposed film

a. Light
b. Clear
c. Black
d. Dark
e. Gray

Identify/Describe

For questions 13 to 17, describe the error that causes the following:

13. Black spots   _____

14. White spots   _____
15. Yellow-brown   _____
stains
16. Cracked or orange   _____
peel appearance
17. Herringbone or tire   _____
track appearance

For questions 18 to 20, circle the correct answer.

18. Too much vertical angulation results in an image that is *elongated / foreshortened.*
19. Too little vertical angulation results in an image that appears *elongated / foreshortened.*
20. A film that has been exposed through its lead foil backing appears *light / dark.*

GLOSSARY

Abrasion The wearing away of tooth structure caused by friction of a foreign object; appears radiolucent.

ADA Case Types The categorization of periodontal disease by the American Academy of Periodontology; four categories have been described: ADA Case Types I, II, III and IV.

Air Bubbles An artifact seen on dental radiographs when air is trapped on the film surface after the film is placed in the processing solution; white spots appear.

Ala-Tragus Line An imaginary line that intersects the ala of the nose and the tragus of the ear; used in positioning a patient for a panoramic film (ala is the tissue that surrounds the nostril; tragus is a cartilaginous projection anterior to the external opening of the ear).

Alveolar Bone The bone that encases and supports the teeth; appears radiopaque.

Alveolar Bone Loss A loss of bone that surrounds and supports the teeth in the maxilla or mandible.

Alveolar Crest The most coronal portion of alveolar bone found between the teeth; it is composed of dense cortical bone and appears radiopaque.

Angle of the Mandible Area of the mandible where the body meets the ramus; appears radiopaque.

Anterior Nasal Spine A sharp projection of the maxilla located at the anterior and inferior portion of the nasal cavity; appears radiopaque.

Articular Eminence A rounded projection of the temporal bone located anterior to the glenoid fossa; appears radiopaque.

Asymptomatic Without symptoms.

Attrition The mechanical wearing down of teeth.

Avulsion The complete displacement of a tooth from alveolar bone.

Benign Harmless or nonmalignant.

Bite-Wing Radiograph A dental radiograph that reveals the crowns of both the maxillary and mandibular teeth on the same film; the primary use of a bite-wing radiograph is to detect interproximal caries.

Buccal Object Rule A localization technique that allows the practitioner to determine the position of superimposed dental structures or foreign objects viewed on a dental radiograph.

Calculus, Subgingival Calculus found below the gingiva; appears radiopaque.

Calculus, Supragingival Calculus found above the gingiva; appears radiopaque.

Canal A tube-like passageway through bone that houses nerves and blood vessels; appears radiolucent.

Cancellous Bone Refers to a lattice-like structure; also known as spongy or trabecular bone; appears radiolucent.

Caries Tooth decay; appears radiolucent.

Cavitation A hole or cavity seen in a tooth as a result of the caries process; appears radiolucent.

Cemento-Enamel Junction (CEJ) The junction between the cementum and enamel of a tooth.

Cervical Burnout A radiolucent artifact seen on a dental radiograph resulting from the differences in densities of adjacent tissues.

Condensing Osteitis A well-circumscribed focal opacity seen below the apex of a nonvital tooth with a history of long-standing pulpitis; appears radiopaque.

Cone-Cut An artifact seen on a dental radiograph when a portion of the film has not been exposed to the x-ray beam; appears as a curved, unexposed radiopaque area.

Contrast The difference in densities between adjacent areas on a radiograph.

Coronoid Notch A scooped-out area of bone located distal to the coronoid process on the ramus of the mandible.

Coronoid Process A marked prominence of bone located on the anterior ramus of the mandible; appears radiopaque.

Cortical Bone The outer layer of bone; appears radiopaque.

Corticated A well-defined outer border of a radiolucent lesion; appears radiopaque.

Cyst A closed, epithelial-lined cavity that contains a liquid or semisolid substance; appears radiolucent.

Density The overall darkness or blackness of a dental radiograph.

Dentin The tooth layer found beneath the enamel and surrounding the pulp cavity; appears radiopaque.

Dentino-Enamel Junction (DEJ) The junction between the dentin and enamel of a tooth.

Developer Cut-off An artifact seen on dental radiographs that results from a low level of developer solution and represents an undeveloped portion of the film; a straight, white border appears on the processed radiograph.

Developer Spots An artifact seen on dental radiographs caused by developer solution coming in contact with the film before processing; dark spots appears on the processed radiograph.

Diagnosis Determination of the cause or nature of a disease.

Diagnosis, Definitive A final diagnosis.

Diagnosis, Differential A list of diagnoses in order of likelihood.

Diatoric A metal retention pin used in anterior porcelain denture teeth; appears radiopaque.

Edentulous Zone An area without teeth.

Elongation A radiographic error resulting from insufficient vertical angulation; the teeth on the film appear longer than their actual length.

Enamel The outer, most radiopaque layer of the crown of a tooth.

External Auditory Meatus A hole or opening in the temporal bone located superior and anterior to the mastoid process; appears radiolucent.

External Oblique Ridge A linear prominence of bone located on the external surface of the body of the mandible; appears radiopaque.

External Resorption A regressive alteration of tooth structure that takes place along the periphery of the root surface.

Extrusion Abnormal displacement of teeth out of bone.

Film Mounting A cardboard or plastic holder used to arrange dental radiographs in anatomic order.

Film Viewing An adequate light source, subdued room lighting and a magnifying glass are necessary in order to view dental radiographs.

Fingernail Artifact An artifact seen on dental radiographs when the film emulsion is damaged by the operator's fingernail during rough handling of the film; results in black, crescent-shaped marks.

Fingerprint Artifact An artifact seen on dental radiographs when the film is touched by fingers contaminated with fluoride or developer solution; results in black fingerprints on the film.

Fixer Cut-off An artifact on radiographs that results from a low level of fixer solution and represents an unfixed portion of the film; a straight, black border appears on the processed radiograph.

Fixer Spots An artifact on radiographs caused by fixer solution coming in contact with the film before processing; light spots appear on the processed radiograph.

Floor of the Nasal Cavity A bony wall formed by the palatal processes of the maxilla and the horizontal processes of the palatine bones; appears radiopaque.

Focal Opacity A term used to describe a well-defined, localized radiopaque lesion.

Focal Trough In panoramic radiography, a three-dimensional curved zone or image layer in which structures are reasonably well defined; a patient must be positioned so that the dental arches are located within the focal trough area.

Fogged Film An artifact seen on dental radiographs when the film appears gray and lacks detail and contrast.

Foramen An opening or hole in bone; appears radiolucent.

Foreshortening A radiographic error resulting from excessive vertical angulation; the teeth on the film appear shorter than their actual length.

Fossa A broad, shallow, scooped-out or depressed area of bone; appears radiolucent.

Fracture The breaking of a part; appears as a thin radiolucent line.

Frankfort Plane The imaginary plane that intersects the orbital rim of the eye and the opening of the ear.

Furcation Involvement A radiolucent area in the furcation of a molar as viewed on a radiograph.

Generalized Occurring evenly throughout.

Genial Tubercles Tiny bumps of bone in the anterior region of the mandible that serve as attachment sites for the genioglossus and geniohyoid muscles; appear radiopaque.

Ghost Image An artifact on dental radiographs produced when an area of increased density is penetrated twice by the x-ray beam; appears radiopaque.

Gingivitis Inflammation of the gingival tissue resulting from the presence of bacterial plaque.

Glenoid Fossa A concave, depressed area of the temporal bone on which the mandibular condyle rests; appears radiolucent.

Glossopharyngeal Air Space An air space on a panoramic film that appears as a radiolucency posterior to the tongue and oral cavity.

Ground-Glass Appearance A term used to describe a radiopacity; refers to a granular, pebbled or pulverized-glass appearance; also referred to as an orange-peel appearance.

Hamulus A small hook-like projection of bone that extends from the medial pterygoid plate of the sphenoid bone; appears radiopaque.

Hard Palate A bony wall that separates the nasal cavity from the oral cavity; appears radiopaque.

Herringbone Pattern An artifact on a radiograph caused by a film being placed backward in the oral cavity; the pattern embossed in the lead foil appears on the radiograph, resulting in a lighter image.

Horizontal Angulation The angulation of the position indicating device (cone) in a horizontal (side-to-side) direction.

Hyoid Bone A horseshoe-shaped bone located at the base of the tongue just below the thyroid cartilage; appears radiopaque.

Hypercementosis An excess deposition of cementum on root surfaces; appears radiopaque.

Incipient Beginning to exist or appear.

Incisive Canal A passageway through bone that extends from the superior foramina of the incisive canal to the incisive foramen; appears radiolucent.

Incisive Foramen An opening or hole in bone located at the midline of the anterior portion of the hard palate directly posterior to the maxillary central incisors; appears radiolucent.

Inferior Border of the Mandible A linear prominence of cortical bone that defines the lower border of the mandible; appears radiopaque.

Inferior Nasal Conchae Wafer-thin curved plates of bone that extend from the lateral walls of the nasal cavity and appear radiopaque.

Infraorbital Foramen A hole or opening in bone found inferior to the border of the orbit; appears radiolucent.

Internal Oblique Ridge A linear prominence of bone located on the internal surface of the mandible that extends downward and forward from the ramus; appears radiopaque.

Internal Resorption A regressive alteration of tooth structure that occurs within the crown or root of a tooth; appears as a radiolucency.

Interpretation, Radiographic An explanation of what is viewed on a radiograph.

Interproximal Between two adjacent surfaces.

Inter-Radicular Between the roots.

Intraosseous Occurring within bone.

Intrusion The abnormal displacement of teeth into bone.

Inverted "Y" A radiographic landmark that represents the intersection of the maxillary sinus and the nasal cavity; appears radiopaque.

Irregular, Expansile Terms used to describe a radiopacity that often represents a malignant condition.

Lamina Dura The wall of the tooth socket that surrounds the root of a tooth; appears radiopaque.

Lateral Fossa A smooth depressed area of the maxilla located between the canine and lateral incisor; appears radiolucent.

Lateral Pterygoid Plate A wing-shaped bony projection of the sphenoid bone located distal to the maxillary tuberosity region; appears radiopaque.

Light Leak The accidental exposure of film to white light; exposed area appears black.

Lingual Foramen An opening or hole in bone located on the internal surface of the mandible near the midline; it is surrounded by the genial tubercles and appears radiolucent.

Lingula A small tongue-shaped projection of bone seen adjacent to the mandibular foramen; appears radiopaque.

Localized Occurring in isolated areas.

Luxation   Abnormal displacement of teeth.

Malignant   A tendency to become progressively worse and, if left untreated, may result in death.

Mandibular Canal   A tube-like passageway through bone in the mandible; appears radiolucent.

Mandibular Condyle   A rounded projection of bone extending from the posterior superior border of the ramus of the mandible; appears radiopaque.

Mandibular Foramen   An opening or hole in bone on the lingual aspect of the ramus of the mandible; appears radiolucent.

Mastoid Process   A marked prominence of bone located posterior and inferior to the temporomandibular joint; appears radiopaque.

Maxillary Sinus   Paired cavities or compartments of bone located within the maxilla; appears radiolucent.

Maxillary Tuberosity   A rounded prominence of bone that extends posterior to the third molar region; appears radiopaque.

Median Palatal Suture   The immovable joint between the two palatine processes of the maxilla; appears radiolucent.

Mental Foramen   An opening or hole in bone located on the external surface of the mandible in the region of the mandibular premolars; appears radiolucent.

Mental Fossa   A scooped-out, depressed area of bone located on the external surface of the anterior mandible; appears radiolucent.

Mental Ridge   A linear prominence of cortical bone located on the external surface of the anterior portion of the mandible; appears radiopaque.

Mesiodens   A small supernumerary (extra) tooth with a conical-shaped crown and a short root located near the midline of the maxilla; the most common supernumerary tooth.

Metallic Restoration   A restoration with a metal component; appears radiopaque.

Microdontia   A developmental anomaly in which one or more teeth in a dentition are smaller than normal.

Midsagittal Plane   The imaginary anterior-posterior plane that divides a structure in half.

Mixed Lucent-Opaque   A term used to describe a lesion that exhibits both a radiolucent and radiopaque component.

Multifocal Confluent   A term used to describe multiple radiopacities that appear to overlap or flow together.

Multilocular   A term used to describe a radiolucent lesion that exhibits multiple compartments.

Mylohyoid Ridge   A linear prominence of bone located on the internal surface of the mandible; appears radiopaque.

Nasal Cavity   A pear-shaped compartment of bone located superior to the maxilla; appears radiolucent.

Nasal Septum   A vertical bony wall or partition that divides the nasal cavity into the right and left nasal fossae; appears radiopaque.

Nasopharyngeal Air Space   An air space viewed on a panoramic film; appears as a diagonal radiolucency superior to the soft palate and uvula.

Neoplasm   A tumor or any new or abnormal growth in which cell multiplication is uncontrolled.

Noncorticated   A term that refers to the periphery of a radiolucent lesion; appears indistinct or ill-defined.

Nonmetallic Restoration   A restoration that does not have a metal component (e.g., composite or acrylic).

Nutrient Canal   A tiny tube-like passageway through bone that houses nerves and blood vessels; appears radiolucent.

Orbit   A bony cavity located in the skull that contains the eyeball; appears radiolucent.

Overdeveloped Film   A dark film that results from excess development time, an inaccurate timer, hot developer solution, an inaccurate thermometer or overactive developer.

Overexposed Film   A dark film that results from excessive exposure time, kilovoltage or milliamperage, or a combination of these factors.

Overlapped Contacts   Overlapped interproximal contacts appear superimposed over each other on a radiograph; results from using incorrect horizontal angulation.

Palatoglossal Air Space   An air space on a panoramic film that appears as a horizontal radiolucency between the hard palate and the tongue.

Panoramic Film   A radiograph that shows a large area of the mandible and maxilla on a single film.

Pathologic Resorption   Resorption of a tooth *not* associated with the normal shedding of deciduous teeth.

Periapical   Around the apex of a tooth.

Periapical Abscess A lesion characterized by a localized collection of pus around the apex of a tooth as a result of pulpal death; appears radiolucent.

Periapical Cyst A lesion characterized by an epithelial-lined cavity or sac located around the apex of a nonvital tooth (also called a radicular cyst); appears radiolucent.

Periapical Granuloma A lesion characterized by a localized mass of granulation tissue around the apex of a nonvital tooth; appears radiolucent.

Pericoronal Around the crown of a tooth.

Periodontal Around a tooth.

Periodontal Abscess A lesion that originates in a soft tissue pocket and is characterized by the accumulation of pus and destruction of bone; appears radiolucent.

Periodontal Disease A group of diseases that affects the tissues found around the tooth.

Periodontal Ligament Space A space that exists between the root of a tooth and the lamina dura; contains connective tissue fibers, blood vessels and lymphatics; appears radiolucent.

Periodontitis Inflammation of the tissues that support the teeth; results in the destruction of the periodontium.

Periodontium The supporting structures of the teeth.

Phalangioma A term used to describe the appearance of a distal phalange of a patient's finger viewed on a radiograph as a result of improper placement technique; appears radiopaque.

Physiologic Resorption Resorption of teeth associated with the normal shedding of deciduous teeth.

Position Indicating Device (PID) The cone portion of the x-ray tubehead.

Process A marked prominence of bone; appears radiopaque.

Pulp Cavity A cavity within a tooth that includes both the pulp chamber and pulp canals; contains blood vessels, nerves and lymphatics; appears radiolucent.

Pulp Stone A dystrophic calcification within the pulp cavity of a tooth; appears radiopaque.

Pulpal Obliteration Total calcification of the pulp cavity within a tooth; appears radiopaque.

Pulpal Sclerosis A diffuse calcification of the pulp

cavity of a tooth that results in a pulp cavity of decreased size; appears radiopaque.

Radicular Cyst See *Periapical Cyst.*

Radiograph An image produced by exposing film to x-radiation and then processing it so that a negative is produced (also called x-ray film).

Radiolucent A black or dark area seen on a radiograph; structures that appear radiolucent lack density and permit the passage of the x-ray beam.

Radiopaque A white or light area on a radiograph; structures that appear radiopaque are dense and resist the passage of the x-ray beam.

Rampant Growing or spreading unchecked.

Reticulation A cracking of the film emulsion that results from a drastic temperature difference between the developer solution and the rinse water.

Ridge A linear prominence of bone; appears radiopaque.

Sclerotic Bone A well-defined focal opacity seen below the apices of vital, noncarious teeth.

Scratch, Film Appears as a radiopaque line on a film; results when the emulsion of a film is removed from its base by a sharp object.

Septum A bony wall that divides a cavity into separate areas; appears radiopaque.

Sinus A hollow space, cavity or recess in bone; appears radiolucent.

Soft Tissue Opacity A well-defined radiopacity located in soft tissue and viewed on a radiograph; a salivary stone or calcified lymph node appears as a soft tissue opacity.

Spine A sharp projection of bone; appears radiopaque.

Static Thin black branching lines seen on a radiograph as a result of static electricity.

Stippled A term used to describe healthy gingiva; refers to the texture of an orange peel.

Styloid Process A pointed, long projection of bone that extends downward from the inferior surface of the temporal bone; appears radiopaque.

Submandibular Fossa A depressed area of bone along the lingual surface of the mandible; appears radiolucent.

Submandibular Shadow An artifact seen on a panoramic film; appears as an area of increased radiolucency below the mandibular posterior teeth.

Superior Foramina of the Incisive Canal   Two tiny openings in bone located on the floor of the nasal cavity; appears radiolucent.

Suture   An immovable joint that represents a line of union between adjoining bones of the skull; appears radiolucent.

Target Lesion   A well-defined, localized radiopacity surrounded by a uniform radiolucent halo.

Transillumination   The use of light to examine anterior teeth for the presence of caries.

Trauma   Injury produced by an external force.

Tubercle   A tiny bump of bone; appears radiopaque.

Tuberosity   A rounded prominence of bone; appears radiopaque.

Tumor   See *Neoplasm*.

Underdeveloped   A light film that results from inadequate development time, an inaccurate timer, cool developer solution, an inaccurate thermometer or depleted developer.

Underexposed Film   A light film that results from inadequate exposure time, kilovoltage, milliamperage, or a combination of these factors.

Unexposed Film   A film that has not been exposed to the x-ray beam; appears clear.

Unilocular   A term used to describe a radiolucent lesion that exhibits one compartment.

Vertical Angulation   The angulation of the positioning indicating device (cone) in a vertical (head-to-toe) direction.

Vertical Bone Loss   Bone loss that occurs in a plane not parallel to the cemento-enamel junctions of adjacent teeth (also called angular bone loss).

X-ray   A beam of energy that has the power to penetrate substances and to record images on film (also called a roentgen ray).

Yellow-Brown Film   A discoloration that results from inadequate fixation or wash time.

Zygoma   The cheek bone; appears as a diffuse radiopaque band posterior to the zygomatic process of the maxilla (also called the zygomatic or malar bone).

Zygomatic Process of the Maxilla   A bony projection of the maxilla that articulates with the zygoma; appears as a J- or U-shaped radiopacity on a maxillary molar periapical film.

ANSWERS TO QUIZZES

CHAPTER 1
1. A
2. Use of fast film, collimated x-ray beam, proper filtration, lead apron and thyroid collar, open-ended lead-lined cones, proper radiographic technique and processing.
3. B
4. D
5. True
6. C, B, A, D
7. C
8. Viewbox with uniform intensity and of adequate size, subdued room lighting, quiet area free of distractions and use of a magnifying glass.
9. Refer to the discussion in Chapter 1 concerning the importance of dental radiographs.

CHAPTER 2

"What Can This Be?"

1. *Appearance:* Unilocular radiolucent lesion with corticated borders.
   Location: Inter-radicular.
   Size: On the original dental radiograph, approximately 5 mm in diameter.
2. *Appearance:* Focal opacity.
   Location: Edentulous zone.
   Size: On the original dental radiograph, approximately 1 cm in diameter.
3. *Appearance:* Unilocular radiolucent lesion with corticated borders.
   Location: Pericoronal.
   Size: On the original dental radiograph, approximately 3-1/2 cm × 2 cm in diameter.

Matching

4. D
5. B
6. E
7. A
8. F
9. G
10. C

CHAPTER 3

Matching

1. B
2. D
3. A
4. C
5. F
6. G
7. H
8. E

"What Can This Be?"

1. Zygomatic process of the maxilla.
2. Floor of the maxillary sinus.
3. Incisive foramen.
4. Coronoid process.
5. Lingual foramen and genial tubercles.
6. Internal oblique ridge.
7. Mandibular canal.
8. Mental foramen.

CHAPTER 4

"What Can This Be?"

1. Answers:
   1. Glenoid fossa.
   2. Mandibular condyle.
   3. Coronoid process.
   4. Maxillary tuberosity.
   5. Infraorbital foramen.
   6. Mental foramen.
   7. Lingual foramen.
   8. Genial tubercles.
   9. Incisive foramen.
   10. Nasal cavity.
   11. Hard palate.
   12. Zygomatic process of the maxilla.
   13. Mylohyoid ridge.
   14. Internal oblique ridge.
   15. External oblique ridge.
2. Answers:
   1. Palatoglossal air space.
   2. Hard palate.
   3. Infraorbital foramen.
   4. Floor of orbit.

5. Zygomatic process of the maxilla.
6. Posterior wall of maxillary sinus.
7. Zygomaticotemporal suture.
8. External auditory meatus.
9. Lateral pterygoid plate.
10. Maxillary tuberosity.
11. Styloid process.
12. Ear.
13. Mandibular canal.
14. Cervical spine.
15. Hyoid bone.
16. Mental foramen.

Matching

3. C
4. E
5. D
6. F
7. H
8. A
9. G
10. B

CHAPTER 5

"What Can This Be?"

1. Amalgam.
2. Gold.
3. Stainless steel crown.
4. Metallic retention pin.
5. Silver point.
6. Earrings.
7. Eyeglasses.
8. The complete denture was not removed from patient's mouth before exposure of the panoramic film.
9. The pit amalgam (labeled) is *buccal*. In the second film (see Fig. 5–58*B*), the tubehead has been shifted down and the pit amalgam has moved up (opposite = buccal).
10. The canine is *buccal*. In the second film (see Fig. 5–59*B*), the tubehead has been shifted down and the canine has moved up (opposite = buccal).

Multiple Choice

11. 3, 4, 1, 2
12. A
13. A
14. D
15. C

Short Answer

16. Gold appears more radiopaque than stainless steel.
17. Silver points appear more radiopaque than gutta percha.
18. Radiographs should be interpreted with the patient present. If questions arise concerning what is seen on a radiograph, examination of the patient can be used to obtain additional information.
19. A localization technique that allows the practitioner to determine whether superimposed structures seen on a dental radiograph are positioned buccally or lingually.

CHAPTER 6

"What Can This Be?"

1. Anterior composite restoration.
2. Cervical burnout.
3. Rampant caries.
4. Root surface caries.
5. Interproximal, moderate.
6. Interproximal, severe.
7. Interproximal, incipient.
8. Occlusal, severe.

Matching

9. D
10. A
11. B
12. C
13. G
14. F
15. E
16. E
17. C
18. A
19. D
20. B

CHAPTER 7

"What Can This Be?"

1. Periodontal abscess.
2. Horizontal, moderate to severe, ADA Case Type III.
3. Horizontal, mild, ADA Case Type II.
4. Horizontal, severe, ADA Case Type IV.
5. Horizontal, mild, ADA Case Type II.
6. Horizontal, severe, ADA Case Type IV.

7. None, none, ADA Case Type I.
8. None, none, ADA Case Type I.

Matching

9. C
10. A
11. D
12. B

Fill In

13. Periodontium.
14. Periodontal.
15. Furcation involvement.
16. Periapical radiograph.
17. Long-cone paralleling technique.
18. Horizontal bone loss.
19. Vertical bone loss.
20. Gingivitis.
21. Periodontal abscess.
22. Radiopaque.
23. Radiolucent.
24. Calculus.
25. Defective restorations.

CHAPTER 8

Matching

1. B
2. E
3. A
4. F
5. D
6. C

Identify/Describe

7. Internal resorption.
8. External resorption.
9. Avulsion.
10. Intrusion.
11. Extrusion.
12. Enlarged.
13. Normal.
14. Atrophic.

"What Can This Be?"

15. Condensing osteitis.
16. Hypercementosis.
17. Periapical radiolucency.
18. Pulp stone.
19. Obliteration of pulp chamber.
20. Periapical radiolucency.

CHAPTER 9

"What Can This Be?"

1. Underexposed, underdeveloped, incorrect molar placement, incorrect placement, crowns cut off.
2. Light leak.
3. Scratched film, incorrect molar placement.
4. No apices.
5. Foreshortening.

Matching

6. E
7. D
8. A
9. C
10. B
11. A
12. D

Identify/Describe

13. Developer spots.
14. Fixer spots.
15. Exhausted chemicals, insufficient rinse time, insufficient fix time.
16. Reticulation.
17. Reversed film.
18. Foreshortened.
19. Elongated.
20. Light.

INDEX

Note: Page numbers in *italics* refer to illustrations; page numbers followed by t refer to tables.